Crops as Sources of Nutrients for Humans

ASA Special Publication Number 48

Proceedings of a symposium
sponsored by Divisions S-4 and C-6
of the Soil Science Society of America,
Crop Science Society of America,
and the American Society of Agronomy
in Anaheim, Calif., 28 Nov.–3 Dec. 1982.

Editorial Committee
R. M. Welch
W. H. Gabelman

Managing Editor
David M. Kral

Assistant Editor
Sherri L. Hawkins

1984
Published by the
SOIL SCIENCE SOCIETY OF AMERICA
CROP SCIENCE SOCIETY OF AMERICA
AMERICAN SOCIETY OF AGRONOMY
677 South Segoe Road
Madison, WI 53711

Cover Design: Julia L. McDermott

Soil Science Society of America
Crop Science Society of America
American Society of Agronomy
677 South Segoe Road, Madison, WI 53711 USA

Library of Congress Catalog Card Number: 84-70717.
Standard Book Number: 0-89118-079-6.

Printed in the United States of America

Contents

Foreword

Because most agronomic research has focused on increased crop yields, the effects of genetic and management variables on plant composition have often been overlooked. Humans, especially those in developing countries, are dependent upon plant products not only for carbohydrate and protein, but also for vitamins, minerals, and essential fatty and amino acids that are critical to a balanced diet and health. Some plant species contain antimetabolic factors, and the bioavailability and usefulness of mineral nutrients in plant products are much affected by plant genotype and mineral availability from the soil. Thus, agronomy, via its various research disciplines, must provide plant products that, when used as food, are nutritious and palatable, and contribute to a balanced diet in a healthy human population.

This publication is a compilation of papers presented at a symposium held at the 1982 annual meetings of the American Society of Agronomy, Crop Science Society of America, and Soil Science Society of America in Anaheim, Calif. It treats the role of plants as nutrient sources, and presents an in depth review of how plant genotype, production practices, soil fertility, and product processing affect the composition in nutritive value of plant products. The material should be valuable to researchers, educators, students, and administrators in charting future actions, and activity for improving plant products as nutrient sources for humans.

We are indebted to the authors for preparing the technical reports, to the members of the organizing and editorial committees for guiding the symposium and developing this publication, and to the staff at Society Headquarters for editing and production.

K. J. Frey
ASA President

W. F. Keim
CSSA President

D. R. Nielsen
SSSA President

Preface

Plant foods are important sources of many nutrients for humans. They contain essential fatty acids, amino acids, carbohydrates, vitamins, and minerals. Yet, the nutrient composition of various food crops is not always optimal to meet the nutritional requirements of humans. Insufficient levels of various nutrients in some food crops, the presence of various "antinutritive" factors, and various processing and refining practices can change the nutritive value of many plant foods. Agronomists and horticulturists generally recognize that crop yields reflect the response of genetic systems to a range of environments, but the associated impacts of these variables on nutritional quality are less well defined. In order to improve the nutritional quality of crops, there is a need for agricultural scientists to be more informed of the concerns and priorities that food scientists and human nutritionists have regarding the factors affecting the quality of these foods. Agricultural scientists should be aware of the potentials that exist for improving the nutritional quality of crops through cultural practices or by breeding. Future developments in genetic engineering may also prove to be a useful means of altering nutritional quality.

This symposium, held on 2 Dec. 1982 at the annual meetings in Anaheim, Calif. is sponsored by Div. S-4 and C-6. It was organized by Dr. Ross M. Welch in response to a request from Dr. David L. Grunes. The information from this symposium should serve as a reference source for students and professionals concerned and interested in improving the nutritional quality of economic crops.

The participants were asked to emphasize general principles. Hopefully "Crops as Sources of Nutrients for Humans" will enhance interdisciplinary efforts which are essential if more nutritious crops are to be bred and produced.

As gross crop yields approach a ceiling, improvements in the nutritional composition of crops should become a more important agricultural strategy.

Editors
R. M. Welch
W. H. Gabelman

Chapter 1

Plants as Sources of Nutrients for People: An Overview[1]

W. H. ALLAWAY[2]

Plants, either consumed directly or by animals and birds to yield meat, milk, and eggs, are an essential food supply. Even in countries where animal products are high in human diets, food products derived directly from plants provide over half of their nutrients. In countries where animal products are scarce, an increasingly large proportion of the nutrients that people eat come from foods of plant origin.

This special publication analyzes some of the problems associated with plants as sources of nutrients for people and will assess some potential routes for improvement of plants for this purpose. The system in which plants capture energy from the sun and take up water and minerals from the soil to form human foods works quite well. This is probably expected because people have undergone many generations of evolutionary adaptation to the nutrients contained in plants. The history of agriculture has been one of increasing the production of those plants known to be useful in our diets.

PLANTS IN HUMAN DIETS

Several features of our diets have an important bearing on the analysis of problems associated with the plants that are used in these diets. First, human diets generally consist of mixtures of different plants, animal

---

[1] Presented at symposium on "Crops as Sources of Nutrients for Humans". Annual meetings, American Society of Agronomy, 2 Dec. 1982, Anaheim, CA.

[2] Senior lecturer, Dep. of Agronomy, Cornell Univ., Ithaca, NY.

products, and sea foods, often in the same meal. The nutritional value of
some nutrients is different when these nutrients are consumed as part of a
mixed diet than when the individual dietary components are consumed
separately. The nutritional status of people is determined by the nutrients
in the mixed diet, and individual components may be a very useful part of
mixed diets even though they contain inadequate levels of one or more important nutrients. A striking example is that plants do not contain vitamin
B_{12}, and any diet composed entirely of plants with no animal products, requires vitamin B_{12} supplementation in order to meet human
requirements. An additional example is the sugar crops. These crops are
processed by refining until they contain only one nutrient—sugar. Even
so they are very useful components of mixed diets and there is relatively
little interest among plant scientists for research directed toward increasing the concentration of nutrients other than sugar in these crops.

Second, the plant components of human diets are, on a dry weight
basis, predominantly the seeds of cereals and pulses, followed in importance by tubers.[3] The seeds of cereals and pulses are frequently processed
by grinding or milling and the seed coats and germ may be removed. In
the case of soybeans (*Glycine max* L.), the protein may be separated from
the oil and these become separate dietary components. The seeds of
cereals and pulses, and the tubers, are nearly always cooked before being
eaten by people. Cooking may change the digestibility of some of the nutrients in plant foods and may also inactivate potentially detrimental
compounds.

Although the dry weights of fruits consumed in our diets are less than
for the cereals and pulses, the fruits make important contributions of certain vitamins. The increased availability of fresh fruits due to the development of refrigeration and products such as frozen citrus concentrates has
unquestionably improved the vitamin C status of people in temperate
latitudes of Europe and North America. The vegetative tissues of plants
generally form a relatively minor amount, especially on a dry weight
basis, of our diets. Nevertheless, the leafy vegetable may contribute important levels of vitamin A, iron, and certain other nutrients.

PLANTS AS SOURCES OF ESSENTIAL MINERALS

Soil and plant scientists have accumulated much information on the
concentration of minerals in the leaves of food crops. Substantially less information exists on the concentration of minerals in the seeds of food
crops, but even so it is obvious that the concentration of minerals in seeds
is less variable than in leaves, and less subject to change from environmental factors such as the fertility level of the soil upon which the food
crop is grown. While the semi-constancy of mineral concentration in
seeds poses some obstacles to the improvement of nutritional quality of
seeds, it also helps to protect people from certain undesirable elements
and compounds. The concentrations of Pb and Cd in the seeds of food

---

[3] More detailed information on the composition of human diets is given in Chapter 2 of this
special publication.

crops is nearly always much lower than in the leaves of these crops. Grains rarely contain significant levels of NO_3-N.

As far as the major mineral nutrients are concerned, cereal grains almost always contain P in concentration adequate for the requirements of people who consume cereals at the average U.S. or world consumption rates. However, cereal grains nearly always contain very low concentrations of Ca. Averaging of values for some of the common cereal foods and common pulses generally indicates that pulses have about five times the Ca concentration of cereals (Adams, 1975).

Phosphorus deficiency in people is quite uncommon, as might be expected from the P concentration in cereals. Possibly Ca deficiency has been common throughout human history and still is prevalent in countries where dairy products are not widely used in diets.

It may be useful to consider whether or not plant scientists should direct efforts toward increasing the Ca concentration in the seeds of cereal crops. Since essentially all the cereal grains are low in Ca it is quite possible that this low Ca concentration in cereals, even the vegetative tissues, is not highly responsive to changes in the level of available Ca in the soil.

In many of the developed countries, dairy products are the major source of Ca in human diets. In the USA, rickets, a Ca deficiency disease of children, has almost disappeared since vitamin D fortified milk became commonly used. The fortification of foods with Ca is inexpensive and safe. All white flour in the United Kingdom is now fortified with $CaCO_3$ (Widdowson, 1979). Even in the developing countries certain food crops are routinely soaked in "lime water" before they are eaten. Calcium carbonate is abundant and is a biologically effective dietary supplement. Decisions concerning research directed toward increasing the Ca concentration of food crops must be weighted against some safe and effective possibilities of achieving the same benefits through food supplementation.

Interest in trace elements in diets and human health has been at a very high level for the past 15 to 20 years. Part of the interest is due to research indicating a number of new trace elements may be essential for animals (Mertz, 1981). The availability of new analytical methods for measurement of low concentrations of some elements in plants and animal tissues has also been a factor. A number of associations between trace element levels in plants and human health have been postulated. Up until recently the relationship between iodine in foods and the occurrence of goiter was considered the only firmly established relationship between human health and the concentration in plants of an element essential for people. The prevalence of goiter was greatly decreased by the use of iodized salt (Underwood, 1977).

When reports of the prevention of "Keshan Disease", a congestive heart failure affecting young children in part of China, by Se supplementation became available, it become evident that one additional soil-plant-human health relationship could be added (Zhu, 1981). People in the Keshan disease area had very low Se concentrations in their blood. These blood Se levels were in the same range as found in animals affected by Se deficiency and were only one-third of those of residents of New Zealand, the next lowest level reported (Robinson and Thomson, 1981). The food supply for the area was primarily locally produced and Se concentrations in wheat (*Triticum aestivum*), rice (*Oryza sativa*), soybeans, and corn (*Zea mays*) were extremely low. Selenium supplementation proved to be so effective in preventing the problem that experiments were discontinued after 2 years and the entire population at risk was provided with supplements, whereupon the disease became very rare.

In large regions in North America both forage and cereal crops are low in Se, although not quite so low as in the Keshan disease area of China. However, residents of the low Se regions of the USA and Canada have over 10 times the blood Se concentration as people in the Keshan disease area of China. The importance of interregional shipments of food in maintenance of Se levels in people in North America is very evident. The hard red wheats, both winter and spring, that are used for bread-making are grown in the Se adequate plains of west central USA and the Prairie Provinces of Canada (Lorenz, 1981). Since bread is perhaps the most common food in North American diets, the contribution of Se from hard wheats grown in the Se adequate regions is probably very important in USA and Canada, and possibly in many other countries that import North American wheat. It is interesting to speculate as to whether or not an unrecognized deficiency of Se in people in North America may have occurred during the period prior to development of food production in the west central part of the continent.

Correction of human deficiencies of Ca, I, and Se illustrate the widely differing solutions that have been effective in compensating for some of the shortcomings of plants as sources of essential minerals for people. Calcium deficiency has been reduced by development of dairying plus effective systems for making dairy products available to a high percentage of the people in certain countries. Iodine deficiency has been reduced by addition of I to salt—a widely used food supplement. In the Keshan disease areas of China, Se deficiency has been reduced by a controlled and carefully regulated Se supplementation of the population at risk. On the other hand, Se deficiency in North America has probably been prevented by interregional shipments of foods. In none of these cases has deliberate change in the food crops themselves been used to decrease the incidence of the human mineral deficiency.

Modification of food crops may, in certain circumstances, be useful in preventing Zn deficiency in people. This deficiency is a problem that has received increasing attention from nutritionists and medical scientists in recent years (Hambidge, 1981). The concentrations of Zn in many normally growing food crops appear to be lower than the dietary levels recommended for farm animals and probably for people. Lean muscle tissue of meat animals is a good source of dietary Zn and probably makes a major input of Zn to diets in many countries. But in countries where meat does not make up a fairly large part of the diet, it appears that a general increase in the Zn concentration in food crops may be desirable. Some recent research indicates that the concentration of digestible Zn in some food crops can be substantially increased by addition of Zn to nutrient cultures, or by Zn fertilization of the soil (Welch et al., 1974; Peck et al., 1980). The levels of added Zn are greater than those required for optimum yield. Zinc concentrations in some crops may be increased through plant breeding programs. But unless the high Zn crops yield more or have other desirable agronomic features, some system of monitoring the Zn in these crops and compensating the growers for producing high Zn crops must be developed if these practices are to be widely adopted. Supplementation of processed foods with inorganic Zn is safe and effective and is being practiced to a limited extent in some countries. When a food processing industry capable of effectively adding Zn supplements to some of the major foods exists, it may be more practical to use this route to improve the Zn status of people than to attempt to increase concentrations of Zn in food crops.

PLANTS AS SOURCES OF ORGANIC NUTRIENTS FOR PEOPLE

Major problems with food plants have been attributed to their lower than desired concentration of protein, inadequate essential amino acid ratios in plant proteins, and low digestibility of the proteins and carbohydrates in plants. Progress and potentials for increasing the levels of protein in plants and for improving essential amino acid ratios in plant proteins are discussed in Chapters 5 and 6 of this special publication. This work will be of most value in countries where the number of different sources of dietary protein is low and just a few food crops, such as cereals, comprise a very large proportion of human diets.

Low digestibility of proteins and carbohydrates is attributed to inhibitors to the digestive enzymes that hydrolyze these compounds. These inhibitors are common in the seeds of cereals and pulses. As is pointed out in Chapter 2, these inhibitors are at least partially inactivated by high temperatures. The seeds of cereals and pulses have for centuries nearly always been cooked before they are eaten. This may be the oldest discovery of a food processing step to improve plants as sources of nutrients.

Total digestibility of any diet is not desirable, except for some very special cases. Many nutritionists feel that it is essential that a fairly large part of the diet pass through the digestive tract regularly for optimum human health. In recent years there have been increased efforts to increase the amount of undigestible fiber in certain diets. The fiber in diets comes primarily from plants. It is quite possible that undigested proteins and complex carbohydrates also contribute to the beneficial effects of fiber in foods derived from plants.

In addition, it should be kept in mind that seeds must have the ability to remain alive but dormant for long periods and then regenerate new plants when conditions for the germination become favorable. If the proteins and carbohydrates in seeds, and especially in the seed coat, were readily hydrolyzed they probably could not maintain this living dormancy and the plant would be at a serious ecological disadvantage in certain climates.

People also depend upon the plants in their diets for several important vitamins. The concentration of some of the important vitamins in plant foods is strongly influenced by storage and processing procedures. Wheat is a good source of thiamine if it is consumed as whole wheat (U.S.

Plant, Soil and Nutrition Laboratory Staff, 1948), but much of the thiamine remains in the bran when the wheat is milled to produce white flour. Potatoes (*Solanum tuberosum*) lose ascorbic acid during storage and during some cooking procedures. Although plant breeders have produced strains of some vegetables that contain enhanced levels of certain vitamins, these new strains cannot exert their full potential in human nutrition unless these vitamins are protected until the vegetables are consumed. The impact of refrigeration and the development of frozen citrus concentrates upon vitamin C intake in some regions has already been mentioned. Vitamin fortification of processed foods is a common practice in the USA and some other countries. So the importance of vitamin levels in plants can vary widely from one country or region to another dependent upon the kind of food processing industry that has been developed.

SUMMARY

Research programs directed toward improvement of plants as sources of nutrients for people need to be designed to fit in with specific systems of food production, transportation, food processing, and dietary customs. In countries where the food supply is abundant and people can choose from many different foods and where a scientifically based food processing industry has been developed, the problems are very different than in some of the developing countries. In order to approach the varied problems and dietary situations that occur in different places, an understanding of all of the factors—environmental, cultural, and genetic that influence the concentration and bioavailability of each nutrient in plants needs to be developed. Soil and plant scientists should monitor the concentration and bioavailability of a number of different nutrients in food crops whenever cultural practices, location of production, and varieties are changed. Food scientists and nutritionists must be made aware of the variations in nutrient concentrations in plants that may result from these factors. For many nutrients "market basket" surveys of the nutrient composition of foods, without information on the variety, place of production and cultural practices, do not give an accurate picture of the ranges in concentration of certain nutrients that may occur. At the same time, soil and plant scientists must be aware of the potential for overcoming the shortcomings of plants as sources of nutrients by food processing and dietary supplements and by introducing new and different foods into our diets.

REFERENCES

1. Adams, C. 1975. Nutritive value of American foods. Agric. Handb. No. 456. USDA.
2. Hambidge, K. M. 1981. Zinc deficiency in man: its origins and effects. Phil. Trans. R. Soc. Lond. B294:129–144.
3. Lorenz, K. 1981. Selenium in U.S. and Canadian wheats and flours. p. 449–453. *In* J. E. Spallholz, J. L. Martin, and H. E. Ganther (ed.) Selenium in biomedicine. AVI Publishing Co., Westport, Conn.
4. Mertz, W. 1981. The essential trace elements. Science 213:1332–1338.

5. Peck, N. H., D. L. Grunes, R. M. Welch, and G. E. McDonald. 1980. Nutritional quality of vegetable crops as affected by phosphorus and zinc fertilizer. Agron. J. 72:528–534.

6. Robinson, M. F., and C. D. Thomas. 1981. Selenium levels in humans vs. environmental sources. p. 283–302. *In* J. E. Spallholz, J. L. Martin, and H. E. Ganther (ed.) Selenium in biomedicine. AVI Publishing Co., Westport, Conn.

7. Underwood, E. J. 1977. Trace elements in human and animal nutrition. 4th ed. Academic Press Inc., New York.

8. U.S. Plant, Soil and Nutrition Laboratory Staff. 1948. Factors affecting the nutritive value of foods. Misc. Publ. No. 664. USDA.

9. Welch, R. M., W. A. House, and W. H. Allaway. 1974. Availability of zinc from pea seed to rats. J. Nutr. 104:733–740.

10. Widdowson, E. M. 1979. Man and the major mineral elements. p. 215–232. *In* K. Blaxter (ed.) Food chains and human nutrition. Applied Science Publishers, Ltd., London.

11. Zhu, L. 1981. Keshan disease. p. 514–517. *In* J. McHowell, J. M. Gawthorne, and C. L. White (ed.) Trace element metabolism in man and animals-4. Aust. Acad. Sci., Canberra.

Chapter 2

Effects of Naturally Occurring Antinutrients on the Nutritive Value of Cereal Grains, Potato Tubers, and Legume Seeds[1]

WILLIAM A. HOUSE AND ROSS M. WELCH[2]

The breadth of the subject matter of this review, naturally occurring antinutrients in plant foods, has forced us to exclude a considerable amount of information. It is beyond the scope of this review to discuss all the antinutrients in the many plant foods that we consume. Rather, discussion here will be limited mainly to a few of the types of antinutritive compounds found in some of the cereal grains, legume seeds, and potato (*Solanum tuberosum* L.) tubers commonly consumed in the USA and Canada. Even within this narrower field of inquiry, no attempt will be made to discuss or review in detail the physiochemical properties of the various antinutritive compounds known to exist in these plant foods. Additionally, discussion concerning the known or proposed physiological functions of the antinutrients in normal plant metabolism will be omitted.

Several recent publications concern antinutrients and toxicants occurring naturally in foods (Ory, 1981; Liener, 1980a; Rosenthal and Janzen, 1979). These publications, each containing excellent review

[1]Presented at symposium on "Crops as Sources of Nutrients for Humans." Annual meetings, American Society of Agronomy, 2 Dec. 1982, Anaheim, CA.

[2]Research animal physiologist and plant physiologist, respectively. U.S. Department of Agriculture, Agricultural Research Service, U.S. Plant, Soil and Nutrition Laboratory, Ithaca, NY.

articles by various contributors, should serve as valuable references for readers interested in more comprehensive information about specific antinutritive factors in foods.

FOOD

General Complexity

Differences among people are myriad and nutritional requirements vary depending on, among other things, physiological development or condition. Nevertheless, a fundamental requirement of all people is that they remain capable of transforming and transporting essential amino acids, essential fatty acids, various cofactors (vitamins and minerals), and energy at a quantity and rate sufficient to maintain the functional integrity of the various cells of the body. Sources of nutrients and energy are the foods and beverages that we eat and drink. For purposes of this review, nutrients are defined as those compounds or elements required for normal development, growth, or maintenance of bodily functions.

Food is the most complex mixture of chemicals to which we are exposed. More than 12 000 compounds have been identified in plants (Reese, 1979), and about 150 different chemical substances have been identified in potato tubers alone (Coon, 1974). Relatively few of these compounds have nutritional significance. In addition to the nutrient compounds, some of the many compounds occurring naturally in plant foods are classified as antinutrients. Antinutrients are compounds or elements that either adversely affect the digestion, absorption, or utilization of a nutrient, or compounds that in some way increase nutrient requirements. Additionally, plants contain compounds called allomones. The latter are nonnutrient compounds produced by one organism that adversely affect another organism (Reese, 1979). Some, but not all, allomones are antinutrients.

Available Foods

In the USA, plants and plant products provide about 58 % of the food we eat (Table 1). A general grouping of plant foods normally consumed by people is shown in Table 2. On a wet-weight (retail-weight) basis, those foods generally considered to be vegetables (leafy, green and yellow vegetables; tomatoes (*Lycopersicon esculentum* Mill.); beets (*Beta vulgaris* L.); pickles; onions (*Allium cepa* L.); cabbage (*Brassica oleracea*); etc.) contribute the most to our diets. This is followed in order by foods derived from cereal grains, fruits, sugars, potatoes, fats and oils, melons and, lastly, foods derived from dried seeds (USDA, 1981). However, on a dry-weight basis, foods derived from cereal grains and legume seeds comprise the bulk of plant foods.

Table 3 shows the percentages of selected nutrients and energy available for consumption from several plant food groups. Major foods of plant

Table 1. Yearly per capita consumption of food in the USA. †

Food group	Amount consumed	
	Retail weight	Percent of total
	kg/person	%
Animal products	269	42
Plant products	371	58
Total	640	100

† Information calculated for the year 1980 from data provided by the USDA (1981).

Table 2. Yearly per capita consumption (retail weight) of plant foods in the USA. †

Food group	Amount consumed
	kg/person
Vegetables	95.5
Flour and cereal products	68.2
Fruits	63.8
Sugars and sweeteners	60.6
Potatoes and sweet potatoes	36.8
Fats and oils	21.4
Melons	9.5
Dry beans, peas, nuts, soy	7.8

† Information calculated for the year 1980 from data provided by the USDA (1981).

Table 3. Energy and selected nutrients provided by major plant foods. †

Food group	Energy	Protein	Fat	Carbohydrate
	% of total available at retail level			
Vegetables	2.7	3.7	0.4	5.1
Flour and cereal products	19.9	18.8	1.3	36.2
Fruits	3.3	1.3	0.4	7.1
Sugars and sweeteners	17.0	<0.05	0.0	38.1
Potatoes and sweet potatoes	2.7	2.3	0.1	5.1
Fats and oils	14.5	<0.1	34.3	<0.05
Dry beans, peas, nuts, soy	3.0	5.5	3.7	2.1
Total of plant foods	63.1	31.6	40.2	93.7

† Information calculated for the year 1980 from data provided by USDA (1981).

origin provide about 60 % of the energy, nearly one-third of the protein, and approximately 40 % of the fat available for intake. More than 90 % of the carbohydrate available for consumption in the USA is provided by the major plant foods. These data (USDA, 1981) are based on the amount of food available at the retail level, and they do not reflect potential waste of food or loss of nutrients during food preparation. Nevertheless, it is readily apparent that foods of plant origin provide substantial amounts of these selected nutrients. However, the total amount of a nutrient in a food does not necessarily reflect the nutritive value of that food. Various factors influence the value of plant foods as sources of nutrients.

Table 4. Factors that influence the value of plant foods as sources of nutrients for humans.

Factor	Example
I. Consumer	
A. Nutritional status	adequate, marginal, deficient
B. Physiological status	age, sex, pregnancy, lactation
C. Disease status	pathogens, parasites, tumors
D. Economic status	quality of food purchased
E. Ethnic background	choice of foods
F. Hereditary factors	inborn errors of metabolism
II. Dietary	
A. Dietary composition	foods eaten
B. Nutrient composition	quantity of nutrients in foods
C. Bioavailability	chemical form of nutrient
D. Antinutritives	protease inhibitors, lectins
E. Nutritive promotors	ascorbate
F. Nutrient interactions	amino acids and trace elements
G. Preparation	raw vs. cooked, refined vs. whole
III. Environmental	
A. Geographical location	soil type
B. Climate	precipitation, temperature
C. Species and varieties	adaptation to factors A & B
D. Plant age	age at harvest
E. Management practices	fertilization
F. Postharvest handling	food quality
G. Processing	milling, extracting
H. Preparation	cooking, soaking

Factors that Affect Food Value

Generally, factors affecting the value of plant foods as sources of nutrients for people can be allotted to one of three broad categories: 1) consumer factors, 2) dietary factors, and 3) environmental factors (Table 4). Some of the consumer factors are age, nutritional status, and disease status. Dietary composition, chemical form of nutrient in diet, bioavailability, and antinutritives are some examples of dietary factors. Examples of environmental factors are geographical location, climate, and various management practices. Additionally, food has powerful sociological and psychological implications. The person responsible for food preparation in the home may select and serve foods based on factors other than nutritional value. Some nonnutritional factors that affect the selection and serving of food are: appearance, ease of preparation, tradition, and to control behavior of consumer.

Although listed separately, many of the factors shown in Table 4 are interrelated and interdependent. For example, geographical location not only affects such things as parent soil material, climate, and species of plants grown, it also may have a bearing on the ethnic background of many individuals living in an area. Ethnic or cultural background may affect the selection of plant foods for consumption. Of particular concern in this review is the effect of selected antinutritive factors on the value of plant foods as sources of our nutrients.

Table 5. Essential amino acids required by human infants and amounts supplied by wheat and soybean proteins.

Amino acid	Amino acid requirements† based on		Amino acids supplied‡	
	Body wt.	Dietary protein	Whole wheat flour	Soybean meal
	mg/kg	mg/g protein	——— mg/g protein ———	
Histidine	33	16	21	33
Isoleucine	83	41	34	50
Leucine	135	68	67	81
Lysine	99	50	24	65
Met + cys	49	25	41	35
Phe + tyr	141	70	75	86
Threonine	68	34	27	37
Tryptophan	21	10	11	15
Valine	92	46	45	51

† NRC, 1980.
‡ Duffus and Slaughter, 1980.

Protein Requirements

Nutrient requirements vary with age, sex, body weight, activity, and environmental conditions. In the USA, values for the recommended dietary allowances (RDA) for many nutrients, including protein, are published by the National Research Council-National Academy of Science. When expressed in relation to body weight, the RDA for protein declines with age. The RDA for protein decreases from about 2 g per kg body weight in infants to about 0.8 g per kg body weight in mature adults (NRC, 1980). Protein requirements may be affected by protein source and by dietary antinutritive factors.

In addition to quantity of protein, the digestibility and quality of the protein must be considered. Plant proteins generally are less digestible than animal proteins. Additionally, when consumed at recommended levels, plant proteins generally have less nutritional value than animal proteins because plant proteins may lack sufficient quantities of one or more of the essential amino acids. Essential amino acids are those that human cells cannot synthesize in sufficient quantity to meet metabolic requirements and, therefore, must be provided in the diet (either in digestible protein or as free amino acids). Lysine is limiting in cereal grains, and the S amino acids are limiting in legume seeds (Duffus and Slaughter, 1980; Pearce et al., 1979).

The amounts of some essential amino acids required by infants, and amounts supplied by wheat (*Triticum aestivum* L.) and soybean (*Glycine max* Merr.) proteins, are shown in Table 5. Mixtures of proteins from cereal grains and legume seeds, particularly soybean protein, can be formulated to meet amino acid requirements. Moreover, soybean protein can provide sufficient amounts of methionine to meet the nutritional requirements of mature humans (Scrimshaw and Young, 1979).

Table 6. Classification scheme for antinutritive substances. †

Group	Nutrient affected	Nutritional effect produced	Substances included
A.	Protein	Depressed digestion or utilization of dietary protein	Protease inhibitors Lectins Polyphenols
B.	Mineral elements	Reduced solubility, absorption, or utilization of element	Phytic acid Oxalic acid Cyanogenic glycosides Thiocyanates Polyphenols Lectins
C.	Vitamins	Increased requirement or inactivation of vitamin	Ascorbic acid oxidase Thiaminase Pyridoxine antagonist

† Gontzea and Sutzescu, 1968.

Amino acids other than lysine and those containing S may become limiting to animals. The sequence in which amino acids in various plant proteins become limiting to some animals has been established. For example, lysine and tryptophan in normal corn (*Zea mays* L.) are colimiting to rats (*Rattus* sp.) (Lewis et al., 1982) and swine (*Sus scrofa*) (Lewis et al., 1979). Threonine is the third-limiting amino acid in corn, and it generally is the second- or third-limiting amino acid in other cereals (Shimada and Cline, 1974; Aw-Yong and Beames, 1975; Jansen, 1977). Knowledge about the order of amino acid limitations of various plant proteins should help in efforts to improve plant protein quality by genetic selection. Additionally, some antinutritive proteins in plants contain high levels of some of the limiting amino acids (Ryan and Pearce, 1978; Pearce et al., 1979); consequently, elimination of these antinutritive compounds from plants may be counterproductive because the levels of various limiting amino acids may be reduced further (Rackis and Gumbmann, 1981).

ANTINUTRIENTS

Classification System

Table 6 shows a generalized scheme for the classification of antinutritives. This system, proposed by Gontzea and Sutzescu (1968), allows for the grouping of antinutritive compounds irrespective of their chemical structure or the mechanism by which they exert their deleterious effects. Although most antinutritive compounds fit the scheme outlined in Table 6, there are many toxic factors that are not antinutritives.

Cereal grains, legume seeds, and potato tubers each contain antinutritive or toxic compounds which may affect the nutritional value of these foods. Some of the antinutrients in cereal grains, legume seeds, and potato tubers are protease inhibitors, lectins and phytic acid. Additionally, various food plants contain vitamin antagonists, tannins, estrogenic substances, goitrogens, flatus factors, amylase inhibitors, and saponins. Potatoes contain toxic glycoalkaloids, but these will not be discussed here. Jadhav and Salunkhe (1975) reviewed some of the factors affecting glycoalkaloid levels in potato tubers.

Table 7. Some antinutrients or biologically active substances found in selected
plant foods or their products. †

Plant		Antinutrient or biologically active substance			
Botanical name	Common name	Trypsin inhibitor	Lectin	Estrogenic activity	Amylase inhibitor‡
		Cereals			
Avena sativa	oats	X		X	X
Hordeum vulgare	barley	X	X	X	X
Oryza sativum	rice	X	X	X	
Secale cereale	rye	X			X
Triticum aestivum	wheat	X	X	X	X
Zea mays	corn	X		X	
		Legumes			
Arachis hypogaea	peanut	X	X	X	
Glycine max	soybean	X	X	X	
Lens esculenta	lentil	X	X		X
Phaseolus vulgaris	beans§	X	X	X	X
Pisum sativum	peas	X	X	X	X
		Tubers			
Solanum tuberosum	potato	X	X	X	X

† References: trypsin inhibitors (Liener and Kakade, 1980; Rackis and Gumbmann, 1981),
Lectins (Jaffe, 1980; Liener, 1979; Liener, 1981), estrogenic substances (Bickoff et al.,
1962; Eldridge, 1982; Liener, 1980b; Naim et al., 1974), and amylase inhibitors
(Buonocore et al., 1977; Jaffe et al., 1974; Knuckles et al., 1976; Liener, 1980b).
‡ Inhibitors of mammalian salivary and/or pancreatic alpha-amylases.
§ Several varieties: kidney, navy, pinto, wax, French and garden beans.

Protease Inhibitors

Several reviews concerning protease inhibitors have been published
recently (Rackis and Gumbmann, 1981; Ryan and Hass, 1981; Wilson,
1981; Liener and Kakade, 1980; Ryan, 1979). Protease inhibitors in soybeans and pulse legumes have been studied more extensively than those in
other plant species. The major protease inhibitors in legume seeds are proteins that interfere with the action of the serine proteases, mainly trypsin
and chymotrypsin, secreted by the pancreas. The protease inhibitor apparently acts like a pseudosubstrate for the protein-digesting enzymes; the
inhibitor binds to the enzyme and forms an inactive enzyme-inhibitor
complex, thus inhibiting the enzyme (Laskowski and Sealock, 1971).
Trypsin, chymotrypsin, carboxypeptidase, and other proteases are inhibited by various protease inhibitors from potato tubers (Ryan and Hass,
1981).

Protease inhibitors have been found in a number of plants. An extensive list of plants containing protease inhibitors, together with the enzymes affected by each inhibitor, is presented in the review by Liener and
Kakade (1980). Some common plant foods with trypsin inhibitor activity
are shown in Table 7. Fortunately, much of the protease inhibitor activity
in most plant foods can be eliminated or markedly reduced by ordinary
cooking and moist-heat treatment. Effects of heat treatment and processing on levels of protease inhibitors in legume seeds and products derived
from legume seeds have been reviewed by Liener and Kakade (1980) and
Rackis and Gumbmann (1981).

Table 8. Effect of heat treatment on trypsin inhibitor (TI) activity in soybean flour. †

Live steam, 100°C	Trypsin inhibitor (TI)	
min	mg TI/g flour	% destroyed
0	50.8	0
1	39.4	23
3	23.7	54
6	14.7	71
9	10.8	79
20	5.3	90
30	4.2	92

† Rackis et al., 1975.

Table 9. Trypsin inhibitor (TI) activity in selected soybean products. †

Product	Trypsin inhibitor activity		
	TI units/mg	mg TI/g	% of raw flour
Soy flour, raw	99.0	52.1	100
Soy concentrate	12.0–26.5	6.3–13.7	12–27
Soy isolate	8.5–20.9	4.4–11.0	9–21
Soy isolate	8.5–20.9	4.4–11.0	9–21
Soy flour, toasted	6.0–15.0	3.2–7.9	6–15

† Rackis and Gumbmann, 1981.

Some typical time-dependent effects of heat treatment on trypsin inhibitor levels in soybean flour are shown in Table 8. In this study, Rackis et al. (1975) determined the destruction of trypsin inhibitor in samples of defatted soybean flour exposed to live steam at 100°C for various periods of time. The process of treating soybean products with live steam is called "toasting." About 79 to 87% of the trypsin inhibitor activity in soybean flour was destroyed by toasting for 9 to 10 min. Additional toasting destroyed more of the inhibitor, but did not further improve the nutritional value of the soy flour.

Levels of trypsin inhibitor found in selected soybean products are shown in Table 9. The amount of trypsin inhibitor in the product appears to decrease with increased processing.

In contrast to legume seeds, potato tubers contain protease inhibitors, particularly inhibitors of carboxypeptidase, that are not readily destroyed by normal cooking methods (boiling, baking, or microwave). Effects of heat treatment on various protease inhibitors obtained from different regions within the potato tuber are discussed by Ryan and Hass (1981) and Huang et al. (1981).

A number of deleterious effects occur in monogastric animals fed either raw legume seeds or seed products that contain high levels of protease inhibitors. As a result of inhibition of proteases secreted by the pancreas, there is increased stimulation of pancreatic enzyme secretion, and chronic stimulation may cause enlargement of the pancreas. Pancreatic hypertrophy induced by protease inhibitors has been observed in animals (chick, rat, mouse) whose pancrease normally weighs more

Table 10. Body weight gain and relative weight of pancreas in rats fed raw soybean meal or purified soybean trypsin inhibitor (TI). †

Diet	Trypsin inhibitor	Body weight gain	Relative pancreas weight
	% in diet	g/35 days	g/100 g BW‡
Casein (10% protein)	--	65.4	0.60
Raw soybean meal§ (10%)	0.40	35.6	0.79
Raw soybean meal§ (17%)	0.68	24.6	0.77
Casein + TI	0.45	40.2	0.74
Casein + TI	0.63	38.4	0.74

† Rackis, 1965.
‡ Body weight.
§ Casein added to maintain dietary protein level at 10%.

than 0.3% of body weight (Liener and Kakade, 1980). Inhibition of the protein-digesting enzymes also results in impaired protein digestion, increased loss of endogenous S-containing amino acids, excessive fecal loss of N and protein, and depressed growth (Rackis and Gumbmann, 1981). Sulfur-containing amino acids of endogenous origin are lost because trypsin and chymotrypsin contain relatively large amounts of these amino acids.

Many of the adverse effects of protease inhibitors have been determined from relatively short-term feeding trials with animals. Feeding raw soybeans or raw soybean flour to swine (Yen et al., 1977; Struthers et al., 1983) or to calves (*Bos* sp.) (Kakade et al., 1976) depressed body weight gain but did not affect the size of the pancreas. When fed to monkeys (*Macaca mulatta*), neither raw soybean flour nor unheated soy protein isolate produced pancreatic enlargement (Struthers et al., 1983). Growth depression, impaired protein utilization, and pancreatic hypertrophy usually are observed in small animals [mice (*Mus* sp.), rats, chicks (*Gallus* sp.)] fed raw legume seeds or purified protease inhibitors. Some results obtained by Rackis (1965) from an experiment with rats fed either soybean meal or purified Kunitz trypsin inhibitor are shown in Table 10. Rackis (1965) estimated that trypsin inhibitors were responsible for 30 to 50% of the growth inhibitory effect of raw soybeans.

Kakade et al. (1973) further studied the extent to which growth depression and pancreatic hypertrophy in rats could be attributed to trypsin inhibitor. These workers fed rats extracts of soybean flour from which the inhibitor had been removed by affinity chromatography. By comparison to results obtained with animals fed the original extract, heated and raw, Kakade et al. (1973) concluded that about 40% of the growth-depressing and about 40% of the pancreatic hypertrophic effects of the original unheated extract could be accounted for by trypsin inhibitors. The remaining 60% of growth inhibition and pancreatic hypertrophic effect of the unheated extract was attributed to the resistance of the native protein in attack by the digestive enzymes.

Trypsin inhibitor levels in soybean seeds (Collins and Sanders, 1976; Bates et al., 1977) and garden beans (*Phaseolus vulgaris* L.) (Wilson, 1981) increased with seed maturation. Reported changes in trypsin-in-

Table 11. Body weight and relative weight of pancreas in rats fed defatted soybean flour (30% of diet) from weaning to adulthood.[†]

Soy treatment	Days fed	Trypsin inhibitor	Body weight	Relative pancreas weight
		mg/100 g diet	g	mg/100 g BW[‡]
Raw	215	1269	432	509
Partly toasted	215	459	498	367
Toasted	215	189	497	364

† Rackis et al., 1979.
‡ Body weight.

hibitor activity during germination vary. Bates et al. (1977) reported that trypsin-inhibitor levels in soybeans germinated for 4 days were about 66% of the level in dry, mature seeds. Using different cultivars of soybeans, Collins and Sanders (1976) observed that soaking (1 day) and germination (3 days) resulted in only about a 13% reduction in trypsin-inhibitor activity in one variety and essentially no change in activity in another variety. The level of trypsin-inhibitor activity in garden beans remained unchanged during the first 5 days of germination, but then began to decline (Wilson, 1981). Bates et al. (1977) fed green mature, dry mature, and sprouted soybeans to rats. Rats fed raw seeds or raw sprouts grew poorly. Cooking the seeds and sprouts markedly improved animal growth.

There are relatively few reports of controlled, long-term feeding trials with protease inhibitors. Some results from one study (Rackis et al., 1979) in which rats were fed either raw, partly toasted, or toasted soybean flour (30% of diet) from weaning to adulthood are shown in Table 11. As in short-term studies, body weight was lower and relative size of pancreas was larger in rats fed raw soybean flour compared to rats fed either the partly toasted or toasted soybean flour. However, continuous ingestion of relatively high levels of trypsin inhibitor (459 mg/100 g diet) in the partly toasted soybean flour did not significantly affect body weight or relative pancreas weight. Previously, Rackis et al. (1975) had determined some biological threshold levels of soybean trypsin inhibitor in rats. These authors reported that destruction of only about 55% of the trypsin-inhibitor activity in soybean flour was sufficient to prevent pancreatic hypertrophy in rats. Consequently, based on studies with rats, long-term consumption of relatively low levels of trypsin inhibitor does not appear to be deleterious. Moreover, neither body weight nor pancreas size was effected in dogs (*Canis* sp.) fed raw soybean meal as 15% of their diet for 16 weeks (Patten et al., 1971). However, Struthers et al. (1983) demonstrated that since the pig, rat, and monkey all responded differently to raw soybean flour, extrapolation of results from one species to another must be done with care. It remains to be determined whether or not prolonged consumption of low levels of trypsin inhibitors have adverse effects in humans. Based on the amount of substances with trypsin-inhibitor activity in various foods consumed in the United Kingdom, Doell et al. (1982) estimated that the daily intake from the average British diet of substances with trypsin-inhibitor activity was 330 mg per person. This amount is equivalent to about 4.1 mg of trypsin inhibitory substances per gram of protein eaten.

For the most part, the nutritional significance of protease inhibitors in nonleguminous plants has not been studied. Ryan and Hass (1981) and Pearce et al. (1979) discussed some of the biochemical and nutritional properties of protease inhibitors in potato tubers. Weight gains of chicks fed autoclaved denatured protease-inhibitor proteins from potato tubers were comparable to control animals, but growth of chicks fed the native-inhibitor proteins was markedly depressed compared to control animals (Pearce et al., 1979). Mitchell et al. (1976) reported that a purified trypsin inhibitor isolated from a strain of *opaque-2* corn did not affect body weight gain, protein efficiency ratio, or weight of pancreas when fed (1060 mg trypsin inhibitor/kg diet) to rats maintained on a 10% casein-diet. The amount of trypsin inhibitor in *opaque-2* corn is nearly double the amount in normal corn (Swartz et al., 1977), so it is possible that trypsin inhibitors in normal corn do not have adverse nutritional effects. Some of the properties of other nonleguminous protease inhibitors are presented by Liener and Kakade (1980).

Most studies concerning trypsin inhibitors, as well as other protease inhibitors, used experimental animals or used nonhuman mammalian enzymes. In a study with humans, Lewis and Taylor (1947) determined that N retention was about 20% lower in two men fed raw soybean flour than when they were fed autoclaved soybean flour. Human trypsin and chymotrypsin have been shown to be inhibited to some degree by soybean and lima bean (*Phaseolus lunatus* L.) protease inhibitors (Coan and Travis, 1971; Figarella et al., 1974; Mallory and Travis, 1975). Krogdahl and Holm (1979) reported that crude soybean extracts and purified protease inhibitors from soybeans and lima beans markedly inhibited the activities of trypsin and chymotrypsin in human pancreatic juice. Wilson (1981) reported that human cationic trypsin was more weakly inhibited by a trypsin inhibitor from soybean, garden bean, and lima bean than was bovine trypsin. The human trypsin reacted with the inhibitors, but the enzyme-inhibitor complex rapidly dissociated. Human anionic trypsin, which represents about 10 to 20% of the total trypsin, reacts more like bovine (*Bus* sp.) trypsin with respect to protease inhibitors. Generally, information is lacking on how protease inhibitors from various plant species affect human protein-digesting enzymes. Such information is needed in order to fully assess the significance of plant protease inhibitors in human nutrition.

Effect of Lectins

Cereal grains, legume seeds, and potato tubers contain proteins that will agglutinate erythrocytes and other types of cells. These proteins are variously referred to as lectins, hemagglutinins, phytoagglutinins, phytohemagglutinins, or mitogens. Lectins have been the subject of several recent reviews (Liener, 1981; Jaffe, 1980; Liener, 1979).

The agglutinating effect of lectins stems from their ability to bind to specific sugar groups on the surface of cell membranes or in glycoproteins; different lectins have different sugar specificites. With few exceptions, lectins are glycoproteins because they contain covalently bound sugars.

Some lectins lacking a carbohydrate group are concancavalin A of jack bean (*Canavalia ensiformis* L.) and those from peanuts (*Arachis hypogaea* L.) and wheat germ (Liener, 1981).

Table 7 shows some common plant foods that contain lectins. Lectins are found mainly in seeds, particularly in legumes, but they also are found in roots, tubers, leaves, and bark (Sharon and Lis, 1972).

Some suggested antinutritional effects of specific lectins in animals include: 1) decreased digestibility of protein, 2) depressed absorption of amino acids, 3) reduced absorption of sugars, 4) growth retardation, and 5) death. Jaffe and coworkers (see Jaffe, 1980) proposed that those lectins with antinutritional significance exerted their adverse effects by causing nonspecific interference with absorption of nutrients from the alimentary tract. The interference with nutrient absorption apparently results from the binding of the lectin to receptor sites on the surface of intestinal epithelial cells.

Growth retardation and death in animals fed raw seeds from several species of legumes are well documented. Some of the growth depression observed in animals fed raw seeds, particularly seeds from several varieties of *Phaseolus vulgaris* L., can be attributed to the effects of lectins (Jaffe and Vega Lette, 1968). Purified lectins from kidney beans inhibited growth and caused death when fed to rats; boiling the lectin extracts destroyed the hemagglutinating activity and eliminated the antinutritional properties of the lectins (Honavar et al., 1962). Kidney bean lectin also depressed the growth of chicks (Wagh et al., 1963), but not to the extent observed in rats. Pusztai and Palmer (1977) reported that kidney bean protein was not toxic to rats after the lectin was removed by affinity chromatography; the purified lectin depressed growth when fed to rats maintained on a casein diet. Lima bean lectin also adversely affects rat growth (Manage et al., 1972).

Although lectins of beans in the genus *Phaseolus* appear to have nutritional significance when they are not destroyed by heat, lectins in some plant species may not be toxic when fed. Soybean lectin probably has little, if any, direct effect on the nutritive value of soybean protein (Turner and Liener, 1975; Liener, 1981). Lectins from peas (*Pisum sativum* L.) and lentils (*Lens* sp.) also may not be toxic (Jaffe, 1980). Moreover, there is little evidence that lectins in potato tubers or those in cereal grains significantly affect the nutritive properties of these foods (Liener, 1981).

Generally, the hemagglutinating ability of lectins is destroyed by moist-heat treatment (Jaffe, 1980; Liener, 1981; Ory et al., 1981); consequently, normal cooking procedures usually eliminate the toxic effects of lectins. However, some lectins are not affected by dry heat. Jaffe (1980) and Liener (1981) discuss some of the conditions under which the toxic effects of lectins might not be destroyed by cooking.

Goitrogenic Compounds

Goitrogenic compounds are found in a number of plant species, including soybeans, peanuts, beans, and lentils (Gontzea and Sutzescu, 1968). Compared to control animals fed casein, Block et al. (1961) observed goiter in rats fed either raw soybean flour, toasted soybean flour, or soy protein isolate; rats fed raw soybean flour had larger thyroids than rats fed toasted soybean flour or soy protein isolate. Thyroid enlargement in rats fed raw soybean flour was prevented by feeding small quantities of supplemental iodine (Block et al., 1961). Konijn et al. (1973) isolated a goitrogenic substance from soybeans that inhibited iodine uptake by the thyroid gland in vivo and in vitro; the authors suggested that the compound was either an oligopeptide composed of two or three amino acids or a glycopeptide composed of one or two amino acids and one molecule of sugar. Beck (1958) suggested that goiter in rats fed raw soybeans resulted partly from increased fecal loss of endogenous thyroid hormone.

The goitrogens in soybeans and other legume seeds probably do not have nutritional significance in humans. Heat treatment abolished much of the goitrogenic activity, and small amounts of iodine supplementation generally were sufficient to overcome the goitrogenic effects observed in animals.

Tannin Compounds

In an extensive review, Singleton (1981) discussed some of the chemical properties and nutritional effects of various phenolic substances of plant origin common in foods. Tannins are plant phenolic compounds with demonstrated adverse nutritional effects in animals. All tannins are polyphenols, and they are potent binders and precipitators of protein. Some physiochemical properties of tannins and their distribution in plants have been reviewed by Swain (1979).

Examples of nutritional effects reported (Singleton, 1981) in animals fed tannins include: 1) decreased food consumption because astringent flavor of tannins makes the diet unpalatable, 2) reduced digestibility of dietary protein because of binding of tannins to proteins, and 3) inhibition of action of digestive enzymes because of binding of tannins to the enzymes. Tannins appear to be toxic to animals when consumed in amounts greater than 1% of diet for extended periods of time. The formation of a tannin-protein complex either before it is eaten or before the tannin reaches sensitive portions of the alimentary tract may ameliorate some of the toxic properties of tannins. Although some varieties of sorghum (*Sorghum vulgare* Pers.) and horsebeans (*Vicia faba* L.) have high tannin levels (Singleton, 1981), the amounts of tannins in foods consumed by people in the USA probably have insignificant nutritional effects. Because of the astringment flavor imparted by tannins, people tend to avoid eating foods with high levels of tannins (Swain, 1979).

Estrogenic Compounds

We included substances with estrogenic activity in our discussion on antinutrients because several of these substances, when fed to animals, depressed body weight gain. Some plant species containing substances exhibiting estrogenic activity (Stob, 1973; Liener, 1980b) are shown in Table 7. Coumestrol and various isoflavonoids are some phenolic compounds that have estrogenic activity.

Knuckles et al. (1976) reported that soybean sprouts contained relatively high levels of coumestrol (71 μg per g fresh wt.), but the coumestrol content of dry soybean seeds, soybean products, garden peas, and kidney beans was low (about 1 μg or less per g dry wt.). No coumestrol was detected in corn protein, safflower meal (*Carthamus tinctorius* L.), or wheat germ.

Isoflavones with estrogenic activity appear to be restricted in their distribution in the plant kingdom, and have been found regularly only in the Leguminosae (Harborne, 1979). Soybeans contain several isoflavone glycosides and their aglycone derivatives. Naim et al. (1974) reported that the isoflavonoid content of whole soybean meal was about 0.25%; about 99% of the isoflavones were present as the glycosides genistin (64%), daidzin (22%), and glyceitein 7-O-β-glycoside (13%). Eldridge (1982) determined that defatted soybean flour contained 0.25% isoflavones; the glycosides and their aglycone derivatives accounted for about 76 and 24% of the isoflavones, respectively. The same isoflavones were found in soybean protein concentrates and isolates, but in decreased amounts (Eldridge, 1982). Isoflavones were not found in commercially produced soybean oil (Naim et al., 1974).

Matrone et al. (1956) reported that weight gains of mice were depressed when each mouse was fed 9 mg of genistin per day. Weight gains of rats were depressed significantly when the animals were fed diets that contained either 0.5% genistin or 0.5% genistein, but weight gains were not affected when the dietary level of either of these isoflavones was 0.1% (Magee, 1963). Based on the data of Naim et al. (1974), Anderson et al. (1979) calculated that a diet containing 19% protein provided by soybean meal would have a genistin plus genistein content of 0.1%. Drane et al. (1980) concluded that soybean meal had estogenic activity; uterine weight was greater in mice fed soybean meal than in those fed the control diet.

Several factors suggest that plant estrogenic compounds probably do not normally affect humans. First, the estrogenic activity of both coumestrol and the isoflavones is extremely low compared to either diethylstilbestrol or to estrone. For example, Bickoff et al. (1962) reported that the relative biological activity of diethylstilbestrol was about 100 000 times greater than that of genistein, and about 2800 times greater than that of coumestrol; however, Kitts et al. (1980) reported that the relative biological activity of diethylstilbestrol was about 100 and 1000 times greater than that of coumestrol and genistein, respectively. Secondly, plant foods commonly consumed by people, particularly soy protein isolates, contain relatively low amounts of estrogenic compounds. Consequently, it is unlikely that people would consume sufficient quantity of these estrogenic substances to cause a physiological or nutritional response (Stob, 1973).

Saponins

Some of the chemical properties and biological effects of various saponins have been reviewed recently (Birk and Peri, 1980; Applebaum and Birk, 1979). Saponins are polycyclic glycosides. They are classified into two major groups, steroidal and triterpenoid, depending on the chemical nature of the aglycone moieties; the aglycones are called sapogenins. Steroidal sapogenins contain 27 carbon atoms, and triterpenoid sapogenins contain 30 carbon atoms. Various sugars have been identified as components of the carbohydrate moiety of saponins. Steroid sapogenins have been studied mainly as precursors for steroid hormone synthesis, and triterpenoid sapogenins have been investigated primarily for potential nutritional effects (Applebaum and Birk, 1979).

Many plant species contain triterpenoid saponins. They have been found in legume seeds, forage legumes, and in some plants consumed as vegetables. Relatively little is known about saponins in many foods and feeds, and different properties that were attributed to saponins have not always been verified (Birk and Peri, 1980). Some of the legume seeds that contain triterpenoid saponins are chick-peas (*Cicer arietinum* L.), horse-beans (*Vicia faba* L.), French beans (*Phaseolus vulgaris* L.), peanuts, garden peas, lentils, and soybeans (Dieckert et al., 1959; Applebaum et al., 1969; Birk and Peri, 1980). Soybean saponins have been studied more extensively than those in other legume seeds used as food, and saponins in alfalfa (*Medicago sativa* L.) appear to have been studied more extensively than those in other legume forage crops.

Some of the biological effects attributed to alfalfa saponins include: hemolysis of erythrocytes, cholesterol precipitation, decreased palatability of diet, and growth retardation in chicks and mice (Birk and Peri, 1980). Reshef et al. (1976) attributed various biological activities of alfalfa saponins mainly to the medicagenic acid content of the triterpenoid sapogenins. Medicagenic acid-type sapogenins contain two carboxylic acid groups, and hederagenin sapogenins contain one carboxylic acid group. Alfalfa saponins that lack acid sapogenins as their aglycones do not lyse erythrocytes.

Soybeans may contain as much as 5% saponins (Pathirana et al., 1981), but soybean saponins lack both medicagenic acid and hederagenin aglycones. Neither food consumption nor body weight gain of either chicks, mice, or rats was affected when these animals were fed very high levels of soybean saponins (Ishaaya et al., 1969). Soybean saponins apparently were not digested in the stomach or small intestine since only integral saponins and no sapogenins were found in the contents of the small intestine of chicks, mice, and rats fed soybean meal (Gestetner et al., 1968). In contrast, only sapogenins were found in the cecum and colon of these animals. Gestetner et al. (1968) demonstrated that the ingested soybean saponins were hydrolyzed by microorganisms in the cecum and colon.

Soybean saponins have hemolytic activity in vitro, but this effect of soybean saponins probably does not have practical physiological or nutritional significance. Neither soybean saponins nor sapogenins appear to be absorbed from the alimentary tract since Gestetner et al. (1968) were unable to find either saponins or sapogenins in the blood of experimental animals fed soybean meal. Additionally, when incubated in vitro, soybean saponins inhibit, to some degree, the activity of proteases. However, prior incubation of soybean saponins with casein or soybean protein counteracts the inhibition of enzyme activity (Applebaum and Birk, 1979).

Soybean saponins probably do not adversely affect humans. In fact, Rackis (1974) indicated that saponins should be removed from the list of antinutritional factors in soybeans. Moreover, Birk and Peri (1980) suggested that since saponins are present in small amounts in many plants commonly ingested by humans, they are probably tolerated by people. Saponins can be extracted from plant materials with hot water or ethanol. Some of the proposed effects of saponins on blood cholesterol levels are discussed in a review by Birk and Peri (1980) and in a recent paper by Pathirana et al. (1981).

Phytic Acid

Phytic acid (myo-inositol hexaphosphoric acid) is the principal form of P in plant seeds, and small amounts are found in potato tubers. Various antinutritional effects have been attributed to phytic acid. It has been proposed that phytate depresses protein digestion, and that it has anti-vitamin D activity (Reese, 1979). As an antinutrient, phytic acid seems to be best known for its affects on mineral availability, particularly Zn. Soluble sodium phytate clearly depresses alimentary absorption of Zn by experimental animals (House et al., 1982), and naturally occurring phytic acid appears to have some effect on availability to animals of Zn in legume seeds (Welch et al., 1974; Welch and House, 1982). Other dietary factors, such as fiber (Kies et al., 1981), may be more important than phytate in determining Zn availability. The role of phytate, and other factors, in mineral metabolism are discussed in another chapter of this publication (Welch and House, 1984) and in a review by O'Dell (1979).

Vitamin Antagonists

Vitamins are conveniently classified into two groups based on their solubility in either fat or water. Substances that either inactivate vitamins or that in some way increase the requirements for specific vitamins in either group are distributed throughout the plant kingdom. Reviews concerning antivitamin compounds in foods have been published (Somogyi, 1973; Liener, 1980b; Klosterman, 1981).

In amounts and forms normally consumed by people, the foods (cereal grains, potato tubers, pulses, and soybeans) considered in this review generally do not contain antivitamin compounds. There are some exceptions, however. Evidence for increased requirements for specific vitamins has been obtained in experimental animals fed some common plant foods or food products. Usually, the need for increased levels of certain vitamins was observed when the animals were fed raw foods.

Under some circumstances, signs of niacin deficiency have been observed in humans and nonruminant animals consuming diets containing high levels of corn. Adding niacin to the diet or replacing corn with other cereal grains eliminated signs of niacin deficiency (Gontzea and Sutzescu, 1968). Substances in corn which interfer with the utilization of niacin and increase the dietary requirement for this vitamin have been reviewed by Gontzea and Sutzescu (1968).

Some vegetables commonly eaten by people have antithiamin activity. Among the legumes, antithiamin activity has been detected in mung beans (*Phaseolus aureus* Roxb.) (Liener, 1980b). Among the cereal grains, a compound in rice bran that is antagonistic toward thiamin has been isolated and partially characterized (De and Chaudhuri, 1976). Generally, neither the chemical nature nor the nutritional significance of the thiamin antagonists in common plant foods is known.

An increased requirement for vitamin B_{12} has been demonstrated in rats fed raw soybean flour (Edelstein and Guggenheim, 1969, 1970a, 1970b). Feeding raw soybean flour to rats increased the turnover of vitamin B_{12} in the body, but it did not affect the alimentary absorption of radioactively labeled vitamin B_{12} administered by gavage (Edelstein and Guggenheim, 1970b). It is doubtful that these observations in rats have significance with respect to human nutrition. Legume seeds generally lack vitamin B_{12}, and vitamin B_{12} from other sources must be provided in diets for humans. Moreover, people normally do not eat raw soybean flour.

Signs of rickets have been observed in turkey poults (Carlson et al., 1964; Thompson et al., 1968), chicks (Jensen and Mraz, 1966), and baby pigs (Miller et al., 1965) fed diets containing either raw soybean meal or unheated, isolated soybean protein. Marked increases in vitamin D supplementation (D_3 fed to birds, D_2 fed to pigs) were necessary to overcome the rachitogenic properties of the raw soybean fractions. The amount of vitamin D required depended on the amount of soybean protein in the diet. The rachitogenic activities exhibited by the soybean fractions were destroyed by autoclaving. Thompson et al. (1968) suggested that the effect of autoclaving was mediated by a pathway different from that involved in the control of rickets by vitamin D supplementation. Phytate has been proposed as the rachitogenic factor (Lepkovsky, 1966), but this has been questioned.

An increased requirement for vitamin E has been reported for chicks, rats, and sheep (*Ovis* sp.) fed raw kidney beans (Hintz and Hogue, 1964, 1970; Hintz et al., 1969; Hogue et al., 1962, 1970). Two antivitamin E factors were identified in kidney beans. One factor was soluble in alcohol and was relatively heat stable, the other factor was heat labile and insoluble in alcohol (Hintz and Hogue, 1964). Some of the effects of raw kidney beans on vitamin E requirements of chicks and sheep were attributed to decreased absorption of vitamin E (Hintz et al., 1969; Hogue et al., 1970). Murillo and Gaunt (1975) isolated an alpha-tocopherol oxidase from alfalfa, soybeans, and beans (unidentified species). When the seeds or flour prepared from the seeds was heated at 100°C, all activity of the enzyme was destroyed. Murillo and Gaunt (1975) suggested that the enzyme was responsible for impaired vitamin E utilization in animals fed raw legume seeds.

The observations concerning increased requirements for vitamins B_{12}, D, and E in animals fed raw legume seeds or seed products probably are not relevent to human nutrition. People normally do not eat raw legume seeds or seed products. Moreover, the vitamin requirements of the animals appeared to be normal when they were fed legume seeds or seed products that had been autoclaved or cooked.

Amylase Inhibitors

The digestion of starch proceeds in two steps. Initially, starch is hy-drolyzed to maltose by the action of salivary and pancreatic α-amylases. Maltose is further degraded by the action of maltases located in the brush-border of intestinal epithelium. Because of changes induced in the starch granule, cooked starch is hydrolyzed more rapidly than raw starch (Snow and O'Dea, 1981). Inhibitors of salivary and pancreatic α-amylases have been found in various legume seeds and cereal grains (Table 7).

Inhibitors of porcine pancreatic amylase were found in 20 species of legume seeds surveyed by Jaffe et al. (1973); the highest levels of amylase inhibitory activity occurred in several varieties of kidney beans. Marshall and Lauda (1975) reported that the kidney bean amylase inhibitor was a glycoprotein that affected human salivary and pancreatic α-amylases. The growth of rats was not affected when they were fed relatively high levels of an α-amylase inhibitor isolated from kidney beans (Savaiano et al., 1977).

Inhibitors of salivary and pancreatic starch-digesting enzymes have been found in several species of cereal grains, including barley (*Hordeum vulgare* L.), oats (*Avena sativa* L.), rye (*Secale cereale* L.), and wheat (Liener, 1980b). Amylase inhibitors obtained from wheat have been isolated from the albumin fraction and separated into three groups based on molecular weight (Saunders and Lang, 1973; Silano et al., 1975; Petrucci et al., 1976; Buonocore et al., 1977). Silano et al. (1975) reported that human salivary and pancreatic amylases were affected to some de-gree by some of the amylase inhibitors obtained from wheat. Lang et al. (1974) reported that wheat amylase inhibitors fed to rats depressed starch utilization, which resulted in reduced growth. An amylase inhibitor from wheat apparently depressed postprandial digestion of raw starch in rats, dogs, and humans; however, inhibitor activity was markedly diminished when rats were fed cooked starch (Puls and Keup, 1973).

Kidney bean amylase inhibitor is rapidly destroyed by heating at 100°C (Marshall and Lauda, 1974), but the wheat inhibitors are more heat-stable and some inhibitory activity persists through the baking pro-cess (Buonocore et al., 1977). Wheat amylase inhibitors are inactivated by autoclaving (Lang et al., 1974), pepsin digestion (Saunders and Lang, 1973), and by trypsin digestion (Puls and Keup, 1973). When consumed in high quantities, some amylase inhibitors may not be destroyed by gastric digestion, and Buonocore et al. (1977) stress that the wheat amylase inhibitors should be excluded from the diet of people in whom digestive proteolysis may be impaired.

Flatulence Factors in Legumes

Flatulence factors in legume seeds do not fit the generalized defini-tion of an antinutritive, but they do cause undesirable responses in people. The flatus causing factors in legume seeds were reviewed recently by Olson et al. (1981). The sugars raffinose and stachyose are largely responsible for flatus caused by consumption of legume seeds (Cristofaro et al., 1974; Rackis, 1975). These sugars are present in amounts ranging from 2 to more than 4% of the dry weight of beans (several varieties of *Phaseolus vulgaris* L.), soybeans, and other legume seeds (Olson et al., 1981). Humans lack the enzymes necessary to digest these sugars, and the sugars are fermented by microorganisms in the large intestine. The fermentation process produces the gases carbon dioxide, hydrogen, and sometimes methane. Any carbohydrate that for any reason escapes digestion and absorption in the small intestine has the capability of causing flatus (Anderson et al., 1979).

Explusion of flatus can be embarrassing, and flatus production has caused headaches, dizziness, nausea, diarrhea, and abdominal cramps and pain (Olson et al., 1981). These effects may result in the omission by some people of legumes from their diet, and thus not utilize a food that is a valuable source of nutrients (Tobin and Carpenter, 1978). Flatus producing factors in soybeans (Anderson et al., 1979) and beans (Olson eta l., 1981) can be reduced by proper processing procedures.

RESEARCH NEEDS

An extensive amount of information concerning specific antinutritive substances in various plant foods has been published. For example, some of the physiochemical properties and biological effects of protease inhibitors in potato tubers are known (Ryan and Hass, 1981), and Hass et al. (1982) recently determined the primary structures of two protease inhibitors isolated from potatoes. Many examples, either of other protease inhibitors or of other types of antinutrients from different foods, could be cited. Nevertheless, we have identified several areas where appropriate research concerning antinutrients might lead to improvement in the nutritional quality of plant foods and be thereby beneficial to human health. These research areas are listed below. Many of the areas mentioned here are interrelated and concern several scientific disciplines. Some of the areas primarily concern either agronomists, plant physiologists, plant geneticists, nutritionists, biochemists, animal scientists, or food scientists. The research needs identified here are not presented in any order of priority.

1. *Function(s) or role(s) of antinutritive compounds in normal plant physiology or metabolism.* Repeatedly, it has been suggested (e.g., Rosenthal and Janzen, 1979) that various secondary plant metabolites (protease inhibitors, lectins, tannins, saponins, etc.) impart resistance against either plant pathogens, insects, or vertebrate herbivores. Additionally, some secondary plant metabolites may function in the control of normal cellular metabolism or cellular differentiation (Jaffe, 1980). The function of secondary compounds in plants needs to be determined or clarified.

2. *Plant breeding programs relative to antinutritive substances.* There is considerable evidence that the levels of specific antinutritive constituents in edible portions of various plants can be either increased or decreased through plant breeding programs. Removal of specific antinutritive substances from a plant might increase the digestibility or availability of specific nutrients. Research is needed, however, to determine whether

or not removal of antinutritives from plants affects various desirable constituents or traits in the plants. Moreover, in the process of selecting plants for increased resistance to various diseases or insect pests, care must be exercised so that new antinutritive substances are not introduced or that the amounts of known antinutrients are not increased to levels deleterious to human health.

3. *Agronomic and management practices relative to antinutrients.* Growing varieties of plants that contain relatively low levels of selected antinutrients is an obvious management practice that affects the nutritional quality of plant foods. Geographical location appears to affect the amount of tannins in barley (Gohl and Thomke, 1976), and the amount of lectins in legumes may be affected by fertilization (Jaffe, 1980). Postharvest handling and storage practices can affect the amount of glycoalkaloids in potato tubers (Jadhav and Salunkhe, 1975). These are a few examples of how agronomic and management practices might affect the levels of antinutrients or toxicants in food. For the most part, however, it is unknown what effects various agronomic and management practices have on antinutrient levels in foods.

4. *Analytical methods and screening techniques.* Development of quantitative methods that rapidly and conveniently measure specific antinutrients in plant foods would benefit plant breeders, food scientists, and human and animal nutritionists. Techniques that could be used to rapidly screen plants for antinutritives would be beneficial to plant breeders. Development or use of standard methods would facilitate comparisons of results among laboratories.

5. *Food processing and preparation procedures.* The activities of some antinutritive substances are markedly reduced or destroyed by processing and heat treatment, but some antinutrients appear to be heat stable (e.g., potato protease inhibitors; Huang et al., 1981). Excessive heat treatment may adversely affect the nutritive value of some proteins. Moreover, plant proteins in general appear to be less digestible than animal proteins (Romero and Ryan, 1978). Research on processing and preparation procedures should be continued to determine conditions for optimal destruction or removal of antinutrients while retaining maximal nutritional quality of food. Research on factors affecting the digestibility of plant proteins is needed.

6. *Mechanism of action of antinutrients, and interactions of antinutrients with various dietary components.* The means by which many antinutritive compounds exert their deleterious effects have been established. For the most part, this information has been obtained from feeding studies with animals or from various types of in vitro studies. In the animal studies, most diets were relatively simple compared to the varied and complex diet consumed by humans. There is some evidence that human and animal protein-digesting enzymes are affected differently by several plant protease inhibitors (Wilson, 1981), but this is debatable (Krogdahl and Holm, 1979). Research on the mechanism of action of different antinutrients should be continued, and possible interactions of antinutrients with other dietary constituents should be explored.

7. *Human health as affected by long-term consumption of low levels of antinutrients.* People normally do not eat plants that are highly poisonous or toxic (Kingsbury, 1964). Moreover, cooking and processing procedures eliminate a considerable amount of the antinutrients in the foods commonly consumed by humans. Nevertheless, low levels of antinutrients are continuously ingested. Eating moderate amounts of a variety of foods reduces the risk of continuous exposure to any particular antinutrient (Coon, 1974). Whether or not exposure to low levels of antinutrients results in less than optimal health remains to be determined. However, studies involving food consumption patterns in relation to human health will be expensive to conduct and difficult to interpret.

SUMMARY AND CONCLUSIONS

Food is a complex mixture of many chemicals. Foods of plant origin comprise about 58 % of the diet of people in the USA. Some of the substances in plant foods are considered to be antinutrients because they interfere with either the digestion, absorption, or utilization of nutrient compounds. A considerable amount of information concerning specific antinutritive substances has been obtained from studies with experimental animals. The significance of many of these antinutritive factors in human nutrition is largely unknown. Some of the antinutritive compounds in plant foods consumed by people in the USA are present in amounts lower than the levels reported to induce adverse effects in experimental animals. Moreover, proper processing and preparation procedures destroy or markedly reduce the activities of some of the antinutritive constituents in several plant foods. Additionally, as indicated by Coon (1974), people generally eat a variety of foods so that the likelihood of continuous exposure to the same potentially hazardous compound is reduced considerably. Consequently, in the form and amounts normally consumed by people in the USA and Canada, the antinutrients in the foods considered here (cereal grains, potato tubers, pulses, and soybeans) probably do not markedly affect the nutritional value of properly prepared foods nor exert adverse biological effects in humans. It is possible that long-term consumption of low levels of antinutritive compounds normally synthesized by plants might have a slow cumulative effect resulting in frank disease or less than optimal health (Liener, 1980c), but this remains to be determined.

Hall (1977) indicated that the key to food safety was variety, moderation, and sanitation. Lack of proper sanitation relative to food is probably a more serious threat to human health than is consumption of low levels of naturally occurring antinutrients in food. Tatini (1981) reported that staphylococcal food poisoning was the leading cause of foodborne illnesses in the USA and Canada. Staphylococcal bacteria are distributed ubiquitously, and they grow rapidly and produce enterotoxins in foods that are mishandled. Similarly, contamination of foods with mycotoxins probably poses a greater threat to human health than does antinutrient compounds. We do not wish to imply that the antinutritive constituents of our diets lack nutritional significance. Rather, we wish to point out that food-borne contaminants and toxicants from several sources may have adverse consequences. Generally, food in the USA and Canada is inexpensive, nutritious, and safe.

REFERENCES

1. Anderson, R. L., J. J. Rackis, and W. H. Tallent. 1979. Biologically active substances in soy products. p. 209–233. In H. L. Wilcke et al. (ed.) Soy protein and human nutrition. Academic Press, Inc., New York.
2. Applebaum, S. W., and Y. Birk. 1979. Saponins. p. 539–566. In G. A. Rosenthal, and D. H. Janzen (ed.) Herbivores. Their interaction with secondary plant metabolites. Academic Press, Inc., New York.
3. ----, S. Marco, and Y. Birk. 1969. Saponins as possible factors of resistance of legume seeds to the attack of insects. J. Agric. Food Chem. 17:618–622.
4. Aw-Yong, L. M., and R. M. Beames. 1975. Threonine as the second limiting amino acid in Peace River barley for growing-finishing pigs and growing rats. Can. J. Anim. Sci. 55:765–783.
5. Bates, R. P., F. W. Knapp, and P. E. Arajo. 1977. Protein quality of green-mature, dry mature and sprouted soybeans. J. Food Sci. 42:271–272.
6. Beck, R. N. 1958. Soy flour and fecal thyroxine loss in rats. Endocrinology 62:587–592.
7. Bickoff, E. M., A. L. Livingston, A. P. Hendrickson, and A. N. Booth. 1962. Relative potencies of several estrogen-like compounds found in forages. Agric. Food Chem. 10: 410–412.
8. Birk, Y., and I. Peri. 1980. Saponins. p. 161–182. In I. E. Liener (ed.) Toxic constituents of plant foodstuffs, 2nd ed. Academic Press, Inc., New York.
9. Block, R. J., R. H. Mandl, H. W. Howard, C. D. Bauer, and D. W. Anderson. 1961. The curative action of iodine on soybean goiter and the changes in the distribution of iodoamino acids in serum and in thyroid gland digests. Arch. Biochem. Biophys. 93: 15–24.
10. Buonocore, V., T. Petrucci, and V. Silano. 1977. Wheat protein inhibitors of α-amylase. Phytochemistry 16:811–820.
11. Carlson, C. W., H.C. Saxena, L. S. Jensen, and J. McGinnis. 1964. Rachitogenic activity of soybean fractions. J. Nutr. 82:507–511.
12. Coan, M. H., and J. Travis. 1971. Interaction of human pancreatic proteinases with naturally occurring proteinase inhibitors. p. 294–298. In H. Fritz, and H. Tschesche (ed.) Proteinase inhibitors. Proc. Int. Res. Conf. Walter de Gruyter, New York.
13. Collins, J. L., and G. G. Sanders. 1976. Changes in trypsin inhibitory activity in some soybean varieties during maturation and germination. J. Food Sci. 41:168–172.
14. Coon, J. M. 1974. Natural food toxicants—a perspective. Nutr. Rev. 32:321–332.
15. Cristofaro, E., F. Mottu, and J. J. Wuhrmann. 1974. Involvement of the raffinose family of oligosaccharides in flatulence. p. 313–336. In H. L. Sipple, and K. N. McNutt (ed.) Sugars in nutrition. Academic Press, Inc., New York.
16. De, B. K., and D. K. Chaudhuri. 1976. Isolation, partial characterisation of antithiamine factor present in rice-bran and its effect on TPP-transketolast system and Staphylococcus aureus. Int. J. Vit. Nutr. Res. 46:154–159.
17. Dieckert, J. W., N. J. Morris, and A. F. Mason. 1959. Saponins of the peanut: isolation of some peanut saponins and their comparison with the soya sapogenols by glass-paper chromatography. Arch. Biochem. Biophys. 82:220–228.
18. Doell, B. H., C. J. Ebden, and C. A. Smith. 1982. Trypsin inhibitor activity of conventional foods which are part of the British diet and some soya products. Qual. Plant-Plant Foods Hum. Nutr. 31:139–150.

19. Drane, H. M., D. S. P. Patterson, B. A. Roberts, and N. Saba. 1980. Oestrogenic activity of soya-bean products. Food Cosmet. Toxicol. 18:425–427.

20. Duffus, D., and C. Slaughter. 1980. Seeds and their uses. John Wiley and Sons, Inc., New York.

21. Edelstein, S., and K. Guggenheim. 1969. Effect of raw soybean flour on vitamin B_{12} requirement of rats. Israel J. Med. Sci. 5:415–417.

22. ----, and ----. 1970a. Causes of the increased requirement for vitamin B_{12} in rats subsisting on an unheated soybean flour diet. J. Nutr. 100:1377–1382.

23. ----, and ----. 1970b. Changes in the metabolism of vitamin B_{12} and methionine in rats fed unheated soybean flour. Brit. J. Nutr. 24:735–740.

24. Eldridge, A. C. 1982. Determination of isoflavones in soybean flours, protein concentrates, and isolates. J. Agric. Food Chem. 30:353–355.

25. Figarella, C., G. A. Negri, and O. Guy. 1974. Studies on inhibition of the two human trypsins. p. 213–222. In H. Fritz et al. (ed.) Proteinase inhibitors. Proc. 2nd Int. Res. Conf. Springer-Verlag, New York.

26. Gestetner, B., Y. Birk, and Y. Tencer. 1968. Soybean saponins. Fate of ingested soybean saponins and the physiological aspect of their hemolytic activity. J. Agric. Food Chem. 16:1031–1035.

27. Gohl, B., and S. Thomke. 1976. Digestibility coefficients and metabolizable energy of barley diets for layers as influenced by geographical area of production. Poult. Sci. 55: 2369–2374.

28. Gontzea, I., and P. Sutzescu. 1968. Natural antinutritive substances in foodstuffs and forages. S. Karger, Basel, Switzerland.

29. Hall, R. L. 1977. Safe at the plate. Nutr. Today 12:6–9, 28–31.

30. Harborne, J. B. 1979. Flavonoid pigments. p. 619–656. In G. A. Rosenthal and D. H. Janzen (ed.) Herbivores. Their interaction with secondary plant metabolites. Academic Press, Inc., New York.

31. Hass, G. M., M. A. Hermodson, C. A. Ryan, and L. Gentry. 1982. Primary structures of two low molecular weight proteinase inhibitors from potatoes. Biochemistry 21: 752–756.

32. Hintz, H. F., and D. E. Hogue. 1964. Kidney beans (Phaseolus vulgaris) and the effectiveness of vitamin E for prevention of nutritional muscular dystrophy in the chick. J. Nutr. 84:283–287.

33. ----, and ----. 1970. Effect of kidney beans, weight gains and unsaturated fat on incidence of liver necrosis in rats. Proc. Soc. Exp. Biol. Med. 133:931–933.

34. ----, ----, and E. F. Walker, Jr. 1969. Effect of kidney beans and taurocholate on serum tocopherol and nutritional muscular dystrophy in chicks. Proc. Soc. Exp. Biol. Med. 131:447–449.

35. Hogue, D. E., G. C. Banerjee, H. F. Hintz, and E. F. Walker, Jr. 1970. Vitamin E and kidney beans in sheep. Fed. Proc. 29:694 (abstr.).

36. ----, J. F. Proctor, R. G. Warner, and J. K. Loosli. 1962. Relation of selenium, vitamin E and an unidentified factor to muscular dystrophy (stiff-lamb or white-muscle disease) in the lamb. J. Anim. Sci. 21:25–29.

37. Honavar, P. M., C. V. Shih, and I. E. Liener. 1962. Inhibition of the growth of rats by purified hemagglutinin fractions isolated from Phaseolus vulgaris. J. Nutr. 77:109–114.

38. House, W. A., R. M. Welch, and D. R. Van Campen. 1982. Effect of phytic acid on the absorption, distribution, and endogenous excretion of zinc in rats. J. Nutr. 112: 941–953.

39. Huang, D. Y., B. G. Swanson, and C. A. Ryan. 1981. Stability of proteinase inhibitors in potato tubers during cooking. J. Food Sci. 46:287–290.

40. Ishaaya, J., Y. Birk, A. Bondi, and Y. Tencer. 1969. Soybean saponins. IX. Studies on their effect on birds, mammals and cold-blooded organisms. J. Sci. Food Agric. 20: 433–436.

41. Jadhav, S. J., and D. K. Salunkhe. 1975. Formation and control of chlorophyll and glycoalkaloids in tubers of Solanum tuberosum L. and evaluation of glycoalkaloid toxicity. p. 307–354. In C. O. Chichester, E. M. Mrak, and G. F. Stewart (ed.) Advances in food research, Vol. 21. Academic Press, Inc., New York.

42. Jaffe, W. G. 1980. Hemagglutinins (lectins). p. 73–102. *In* I. E. Liener (ed.) Toxic constituents of plant foodstuffs. 2nd ed. Academic Press, Inc., New York.

43. ----, and C. L. Vega Lette. 1968. Heat-labile growth-inhibiting factors in beans. J. Nutr. 94:203–210.

44. ----, R. Moreno, and V. Wallis. 1973. Amylase inhibitors in legume seeds. Nutr. Rep. Int. 7:169–174.

45. Jansen, G. R. 1977. Amino acid fortification. p. 177–203. *In* C. E. Bodwell (ed.) Evaluation of proteins for humans. AVI Publishing Co., Westport, Conn.

46. Jensen, L. S., and F. R. Mraz. 1966. Rachitogenic activity of isolated soy protein for chicks. J. Nutr. 88:249–253.

47. Kakade, M. L., D. E. Hoffa, and I. E. Liener. 1973. Contribution of trypsin inhibitors to the deleterious effects of unheated soybeans fed to rats. J. Nutr. 103:1772–1778.

48. ----, R. D. Thompson, W. E. Englestad, G. C. Behrens, R. D. Yoder, and F. M. Crane. 1976. Failure of soybean trypsin inhibitor to exert deleterious effects in calves. J. Dairy Sci. 59:1484–1489.

49. Kies, D., D. Beshgetoor, and H. M. Fox. 1981. Dietary fiber and zinc bioavailability for humans. p. 319–329. *In* R. L. Ory (ed.) Antinutrients and natural toxicants in foods. Food and Nutrition Press, Inc., Westport, Conn.

50. Kingsbury, J. M. 1964. Poisonous plants of the United States and Canada. Prentice-Hall, Englewood Cliffs, N.J.

51. Kitts, D. D., C. R. Krishnamurti, and W. D. Kitts. 1980. Uterine weight changes and ^{3}H-uridine uptake in rats with phytoestrogens. Can. J. Anim. Sci. 60:531–534.

52. Klosterman, H. J. 1981. Vitamin B_6 antagonists in natural products. p. 295–317. *In* R. L. Ory (ed.) Antinutrients and natural toxicants in foods. Food and Nutrition Press, Inc., Westport, Conn.

53. Knuckles, B. E., D. de Fremery, and G. O. Kohler. 1976. Coumestrol content of fractions obtained during wet processing of alfalfa. J. Agric. Food Chem. 24:1177–1180.

54. Konijn, A. M., B. Gershon, and K. Guggenheim. 1973. Further purification and mode of action of a goitrogenic material from soybean flour. J. Nutr. 103:378–383.

55. Krogdahl, A., and H. Holm. 1979. Inhibition of human and rat pancreatic proteinases by crude and purified soybean proteinase inhibitors. J. Nutr. 109:551–558.

56. Lang, J. A., L. E. Chang-Hum, P. S. Reyes, and G. M. Briggs. 1974. Interference of starch metabolism by α-amylase inhibitors. Fed. Proc. 33:718 (abstr.).

57. Laskowski, Jr., M., I. Kato, T. R. Leary, J. Schroede, and R. W. Sealock. 1974. Evolution of specificity of protein proteinase inhibitors. p. 597–611. *In* H. Fritz et al. (ed.) Proteinase inhibitors. Proc. 2nd Int. Res. Conf. Springer-Verlag, New York.

58. ----, and R. W. Sealock. 1971. Protein proteinase inhibitors—molecular aspects. The Enzymes 3:376–473.

59. Lepkovsky, S. 1966. Antivitamins in foods. p. 98–104. *In* Food Protection Committee (ed.) Toxicants occurring naturally in foods. Public. 1354, Natl. Res. Council, Natl. Acad. Sci., Washington, D.C.

60. Lewis, A. H., M. B. Barnes, D. A. Grosbach, and E. R. Peo, Jr. 1982. Sequence in which the amino acids of corn (*Zea mays*) become limiting for growing rats. J. Nutr. 112:782–788.

61. Lewis, A. J., E. R. Peo, Jr., B. D. Moser, and T. D. Crenshaw. 1979. Additions of lysine, tryptophan, methionine and isoleucine to all-corn diets for finishing swine. Nutr. Rep. Int. 19:533–540.

62. Lewis, J. H., and F. H. L. Taylor. 1947. Comparative utilization of raw and autoclaved soy bean protein by the human. Proc. Soc. Exp. Biol. Med. 64:85–87.

63. Liener, I. E. 1979. Phytohemagglutinins. p. 567–598. *In* G. A. Rosenthal, and D. H. Janzen (ed.) Herbivores. Their interaction with secondary plant metabolites. Academic Press, Inc., New York.

64. ----. 1980a. Toxic constituents of plant foodstuffs. 2nd ed. Academic Press, Inc., New York.

65. ----. 1980b. Miscellaneous toxic factors. p. 429–467. *In* I. E. Liener (ed.) Toxic constituents of plant foodstuffs. 2nd ed. Academic Press, Inc., New York.

66. ————. 1980c. Introduction. p. 1–5. *In* I. E. Liener (ed.) Toxic constituents of plant foodstuffs, 2nd ed. Academic Press, Inc., New York.

67. ————. 1981. The nutritional significance of the plant lectins. p. 143–157. *In* R. L. Ory (ed.) Antinutrients and natural toxicants in foods. Food and Nutrition Press, Inc., Westport, Conn.

68. ————, and M. L. Kakade. 1980. Protease inhibitors. p. 7–71. *In* I. E. Liener (ed.) Toxic constituents of plant foodstuffs. 2nd ed. Academic Press, Inc., New York.

69. Magee, A. C. 1963. Biological responses of young rats fed diets containing genistin and genistein. J. Nutr. 80:151–156.

70. Mallory, P. A., and J. Travis. 1975. Inhibition spectra of the human pancreatic endopeptidases. Am. J. Clin. Nutr. 28:823–830.

71. Manage, L., A. Joshi, and K. Sohonie. 1972. Toxicity to rats and mice of purified phytohemagglutinins from four Indian legumes. Toxicon 10:89–91.

72. Marshall, J. J., and C. M. Lauda. 1975. Purification and properties of phaseolamin, an inhibitor of α-amylase, from kidney bean, *Phaseolus vulgaris*. J. Biol. Chem. 250:8030–8037.

73. Matrone, G., W. W. G. Smart, Jr., M. W. Carter, and V. W. Smart. 1956. Effect of genistin on growth and development of the male mouse. J. Nutr. 59:235–241.

74. Miller, E. R., D. E. Ullrey, C. L. Zutaut, J. A. Hoefer, and R. L. Leucke. 1965. Comparisons of casein and soy proteins upon mineral balance and vitamin D_2 requirement of the baby pig. J. Nutr. 85:347–354.

75. Mitchell, H. L., D. B. Parrish, M. Corney, and C. E. Wassom. 1976. Effects of corn trypsin inhibitor on growth of rats. J. Agric. Food Chem. 24:1254–1255.

76. Murillo, E., and J. K. Gaunt. 1975. Investigations on alfa-tocopherol oxidase in beans, alfalfa and soybeans. 1st Chem. Congr. North Am. Continent, BMPS Abstr. No. 155.

77. Naim, M., B. Gestetner, S. Zilkah, Y. Birk, and A. Bondi. 1974. Soybean isoflavones. Characterization, determination, and antifungal activity. J. Agric. Food Chem. 22:806–810.

78. National Research Council, Food and Nutrition Board. 1980. Recommended dietary allowances. 9th ed. Natl. Acad. Sci., Washington, D.C.

79. O'Dell, B. L. 1979. Effect of soy protein on trace mineral availability. p. 187–204. *In* H. L. Wilcke, D. T. Hopkins, and D. H. Waggle (ed.) Soy protein and human nutrition. Academic Press, Inc., New York.

80. Olson, A. C., G. M. Gray, M. R. Gumbmann, C. R. Sell, and J. R. Wagner. 1981. Flatus causing factors in legumes. p. 275–294. *In* R. L. Ory (ed.) Antinutrients and natural toxicants in foods. Food and Nutrition Press, Inc., Westport, Conn.

81. Ory, R. L. 1981. Antinutrients and natural toxicants in foods. Food and Nutrition Press, Inc., Westport, Conn.

82. ————, T. C. Bog-Hansen, and R. R. Mod. 1981. Properties of hemagglutinins in rice and other cereal grains. p. 159–168. *In* R. L. Ory (ed.) Antinutrients and natural toxicants in foods. Food and Nutrition Press, Inc., Westport, Conn.

83. Pathirana, C., M. J. Gibney, and T. G. Taylor. 1981. The effect of dietary protein source and saponins on serum lipids and the excretion of bile acids and neutral sterols in rabbits. Brit. J. Nutr. 46:421–430.

84. Patten, J. R., E. A. Richards, and J. Wheeler. 1971. The effect of raw soybean on the pancreases of adult dogs. Proc. Soc. Exp. Biol. Med. 137:59–63.

85. Pearce, G., J. McGinnis, and C. A. Ryan. 1979. Utilization by chicks of half-cystine from native and denatured proteinase inhibitor proteins. Proc. Soc. Exp. Biol. Med. 160:180–184.

86. Petrucci, T., A. Rab, M. Tomasi, and V. Silano. 1976. Further characterization studies of the α-amylase protein inhibitor of gel electrophoretic mobility 0.19 from the wheat kernel. Biochim. Biophys. Acta 420:288–297.

87. Puls, W., and U. Keup. 1973. Influence of an α-amylase inhibitor (BAY d 7791) on blood glucose, serum insulin and NEFA in starch loading tests in rats, dogs and man. Diabetologia 9:97–101.

88. Pusztai, A., and R. Palmer. 1977. Nutritional evaluation of kidney beans (*Phaseolus vulgaris*): the toxic principle. J. Sci. Food Agric. 28:620–623.

89. Rackis, J. J. 1965. Physiological properties of soybean trypsin inhibitor and their relationship to pancreatic hypertrophy and growth inhibition of rats. Fed. Proc. 24:1488–1493.

90. ————. 1974. Biological and physiological factors in soybeans. J. Am. Oil Chem. Soc. 51: 161A–174A.

91. ————. 1975. Oligosaccharides in food legumes: alpha-galactosidase activity and the flatus problem. p. 207–222. In A. Jeanes, and J. Hodge (ed.) Physiological effects of food carbohydrates. ACS Symp. Series No. 15, Am. Chem. Soc., Washington, D.C.

92. ————, and M. R. Gumbmann. 1981. Protease inhibitors: physiological properteis and nutritional significance. p. 203–237. In R. L. Ory (ed.) Antinutrients and natural toxicants in foods. Food and Nutrition Press, Inc., Westport, Conn.

93. ————, J. E. McGhee, and A. N. Booth. 1975. Biological threshold levels of soybean trypsin inhibitors by rat bioassays. Cereal Chem. 52:85–92.

94. ————, ————, M. R. Gumbmann, and A. N. Booth. 1979. Effects of soy proteins containing trypsin inhibitors on long-term feeding studies in rats. J. Am. Oil Chem. Soc. 56: 162–168.

95. Reese, J. C. 1979. Interactions of allelochemicals with nutrients in herbivore food. p. 309–330. In G. A. Rosenthal, and D. H. Janzen (ed.) Herbivores. Their interaction with secondary plant metabolites. Academic Press, Inc., New York.

96. Reshef, G., B. Gestetner, Y. Birk, and A. Bondi. 1976. Effect of alfalfa saponins on the growth and some aspects of lipid metabolism of mice and quails. J. Sci. Food Agric. 27: 63–72.

97. Romero, J., and D. S. Ryan. 1978. Susceptibility of the major storage protein of the bean, *Phaseolus vulgaris* L., to in vitro enzymatic hydrolysis. J. Agric. Food Chem. 26: 784–788.

98. Rosenthal, G. A., and D. H. Janzen. 1979. Herbivores. Their interaction with secondary plant metabolites. Academic Press, Inc., New York.

99. Ryan, C. A. 1979. Proteinase inhibitors. p. 599–618. In G. A. Rosenthal, and D. H. Janzen (ed.) Herbivores. Their interaction with secondary plant metabolites. Academic Press, Inc., New York.

100. ————, and G. M. Hass. 1981. Structural, evolutionary and nutritional properties of proteinase inhibitors from potatoes. p. 169–185. In R. L. Ory (ed.) Antinutrients and natural toxicants in foods. Food and Nutrition Press, Inc., Westport, Conn.

101. ————, and G. Pearce. 1978. Proteinase inhibitor proteins as genetic markers for identifying high protein potato clones. Am. Potato J. 55:351–358.

102. Saunders, R. M., and J. A. Lang. 1973. α-Amylase inhibitors in *Triticum aestivum*: purification and physical-chemical properties. Phytochemistry 12:1237–1241.

103. Savaiano, D. A., J. R. Powers, M. J. Costello, J. R. Whitaker, and A. J. Clifford. 1977. The effect of an α-amylase inhibitor on the growth rate of weanling rats. Nutr. Rep. Int. 15:443–449.

104. Scrimshaw, N. S., and V. R. Young. 1979. Soy protein in adult human nutrition: a review with new data. p. 121–143. In H. L. Wilcke, D. T. Hopkins, and D. H. Waggle (ed.) Soy protein and human nutrition. Academic Press, Inc., New York.

105. Sharon, N., and H. Lis. 1972. Lectins: cell-agglutinating and sugar-specific proteins. Science 177:949–959.

106. Shimada, A., and T. R. Cline. 1974. Limiting amino acids of triticale for the growing rat and pig. J. Anim. Sci. 38:941–946.

107. Silano, V., M. Furia, L. Gianfreda, A. Macri, R. Palescandolo, A. Rab, V. Scardi, E. Stella, and F. Valfre. 1975. Inhibition of amylases from different origins by albumins from the wheat kernel. Biochim. Biophys. Acta 391:170–178.

108. Singleton, V. L. 1981. Naturally occurring food toxicants: phenolic substances of plant origin common in foods. p. 149–242. In C. O. Chichester et al. (ed.) Advances in food research, Vol. 27. Academic Press, Inc., New York.

109. Somogyi, J. C. 1973. Antivitamins. p. 254–275. In National Research Council, Food Protection Committee (ed.) Toxicants occurring naturally in foods. 2nd ed. Natl. Res. Council, Natl. Acad. Sci., Washington, D.C.

110. Snow, P., and K. O'Dea. 1981. Factors affecting the rate of hydrolysis of starch in food. Am. J. Clin. Nutr. 34:2721–2727.

111. Stob, M. 1973. Estogens in food. p. 550–557. *In* National Research Council, Food Protection Committee (ed.) Toxicants occurring naturally in foods. 2nd ed. Natl. Res. Council, Natl. Acad. Sci., Washington, D.C.

112. Struthers, B. J., J. R. MacDonald, R. R. Dahlgren, and D. T. Hopkins. 1983. Effects on the monkey, pig and rat pancreas of soy products with varying levels of trypsin inhibitor and comparison with the administration of cholecystokinin. J. Nutr. 113:86–97.

113. Swain, T. 1979. Tannins and lignins. p. 657–682. *In* G. A. Rosenthal, and D. H. Janzen (ed.) Herbivores. Their interaction with secondary plant metabolites. Academic Press, Inc., New York.

114. Swartz, M. J., H. L. Mitchell, D. J. Cox, and G. R. Reeck. 1977. Isolation and characterization of trypsin inhibitor from opaque-2 corn seeds. J. Biol. Chem. 252:8105–8107.

115. Tatini, S. R. 1981. Thermonuclease as an indicator of staphylococcal enterotoxins in food. p. 53–75. *In* R. L. Ory (ed.) Antinutrients and natural toxicants in foods. Food and Nutrition Press, Inc., Westport, Conn.

116. Thompson, O. J., C. W. Carlson, I. S. Palmer, and O. E. Olson. 1968. Destruction of rachitogenic activity of isolated soybean protein by autoclaving as demonstrated with turkey poults. J. Nutr. 94:227–232.

117. Tobin, G., and K. J. Carpenter. 1978. The nutritional value of the dry bean (*Phaseolus vulgaris*): a literature review. Nutr. Abstr. Rev. 48:919–936.

118. Turner, R. H., and I. E. Liener. 1975. The effect of selective removal of hemagglutinins on the nutritive value of soybeans. J. Agric. Food. Chem. 23:481–487.

119. U.S. Department of Agriculture. 1981. Agricultural statistics. U.S. Government Printing Office, Washington, D.C.

120. Wagh, P. V., D. F. Klaustermeier, P. E. Waibel, and I. E. Liener. 1963. Nutritive value of red kidney beans (*Phaseolus vulgaris*) for chicks. J. Nutr. 80:191–195.

121. Welch, R. M., and W. A. House. 1982. Availability to rats of zinc from soybean seeds as affected by maturity of seed, source of dietary protein, and soluble phytate. J. Nutr. 112:879–885.

122. ————, and ————. 1984. Factors affecting the bioavailability of mineral nutrients in plant foods. p. 37–54. *In* R. M. Welch and W. H. Gabelman (ed.) Crops as sources of nutrients for humans. Am. Soc. of Agron., Crop Sci. Soc. of Am., and Soil Sci. Soc. of Am. Spec. Pub. no. 48. Am. Soc. of Agron., Madison, Wis.

123. ————, ————, and W. H. Allaway. 1974. Availability of zinc from pea seeds to rats. J. Nutr. 104:733–740.

124. Wilson, K. A. 1981. The structure, function, and evolution of legume proteinase inhibitors. p. 187–202. *In* R. L. Ory (ed.) Antinutrients and natural toxicants in foods. Food and Nutrition Press, Inc., Westport, Conn.

125. Yen, J. T., A. H. Jensen, and J. Simon. 1977. Effect of dietary raw soybean and soybean trypsin inhibitor on trypsin and chymotrypsin activities in the pancreas and in small intestinal juice of growing swine. J. Nutr. 107:156–165.

Chapter 3

Factors Affecting the Bioavailability of Mineral Nutrients in Plant Foods[1]

ROSS M. WELCH AND WILLIAM A. HOUSE[2]

When essential mineral nutrients move from soils to plants to animals and humans, there occurs selectivity for, and barriers to, the transfer from lower to higher trophic levels. The idea of mineral nutrient bioavailability was conceived to deal with the inefficient transfer of mineral nutrients at various levels in the food web. Bioavailability to organisms of a mineral element is that proportion of an element in a nutrient medium which is potentially absorbable in a form which is metabolically active. The concept of bioavailability is routinely used by agronomists and soil scientists involved in soil fertility studies. In these studies the amounts of elements that are available, rather than total mineral nutrient content, are of primary importance in determining the adequacy of soil nutrients required for optimum plant growth. Similarly, the concept of bioavailability is important when considering the mineral nutrient content of edible plants as sources of essential elements for humans. The total amount of a mineral nutrient in a food does not necessarily reflect the nutritional quality of that food. The nutritional quality of plant foods, with respect to minerals, is determined by the proportion of absorbable and utilizable essential elements in a meal (Mertz, 1980; Quarterman, 1973). Some plant foods may contain factors (e.g., compounds or elements) that

---

[1] Presented at symposium on "Crops as Sources of Nutrients for Humans". Annual meetings, Am. Soc. of Agron., 2 Dec. 1982, Anaheim, CA.

[2] Plant physiologist and research animal physiologist, USDA, ARS, U.S. Plant, Soil and Nutrition Laboratory, Ithaca, NY.

---

affect absorption and/or utilization of elements either by enhancing or diminishing their effectiveness (Davies, 1979; Gontzea and Sutzescu, 1968). Although human mineral deficiency diseases frequently result from low dietary intakes of minerals, such diseases may occur when dietary mineral levels are within ranges normally considered adequate (Bremner and Mills, 1981). The latter circumstances can occur when physiological or genetic variables decrease the bioavailability of mineral elements.

Because most of the processes and factors that affect mineral nutrient bioavailability are not understood, predicting the available mineral nutrient content of food crops is currently extremely difficult, if not impossible. This chapter presents some reasons for increased interest in, and some factors affecting, mineral nutrient bioavailability in plant foods. Consideration is also given to areas of knowledge in which nutritional research must be expanded before plant scientists can affect significant improvements in bioavailability of mineral nutrients in plant foods. Suggestions as to what currently can be done by agriculturalists to improve food crops as sources of mineral nutrients will be discussed, along with examples of research supporting these suggestions. Finally, research areas in the soil and plant sciences where lack of knowledge is limiting progress toward improving food crops as sources of mineral nutrients will be explored. Several references are available for those readers interested in more detailed discussions of the bioavailability of mineral nutrients (e.g., Ammerman and Miller, 1972; Beeson et al., 1978; Bremner and Mills, 1981; Chesters, 1976; Davies, 1979; Fritz, 1973; Goodhart and Shils, 1980; Harper, 1976; Mertz, 1981a; Quarterman, 1973; Underwood, 1977; Widdowson, 1980).

Interest in improving crops as sources of mineral nutrients for humans is not new. The need for improvement is taking on increasing importance (Mertz, 1980, 1981a, 1981b; Underwood, 1981). Nutritionists are becoming increasingly aware of the role edible plant products can play in the nutritional health of people worldwide.

Subtle mineral nutrient deficiencies may cause marginal or subclinical impairment of human health and productivity. These deficiencies may occur more frequently because of: 1) trends towards intensive agricultural practices to produce maximum yields on soils of marginal trace element status; and 2) changing agricultural systems towards monoculture type practices. These agricultural practices may increase the rate of depletion of certain nutritionally important trace elements from poorer soil types (Allaway, 1968; Beeson and Matrone, 1976; Kubota and Allaway, 1972; Mertz, 1980, 1981b). Some of the "newer" recently discovered trace elements essential for animals seem especially important in this regard. These include elements such as Se, V, Sn, Cr, and As (see Table 1). Apparently normal, high-yielding plants could be produced on soils depleted of some of these trace elements that are essential to animals but not for plants (Allaway, 1968; Mertz, 1981b). Further, as animal proteins become more expensive and less available, per capita consumption of plant foods will increase. Therefore, their importance as sources of essential nutrients for humans should increase.

Table 1. Micronutrients and trace elements required by higher plants and/or animals. †

Element	Essentiality for higher plants	Essentiality for animals
Na‡	?	+
Fe	+	+
Cu	+	+
Zn	+	+
Mn	+	+
Cl	+	+
B	+	?
Mo	+	?
F	0	+
Si	?	+
V	0	+
Cr	0	+
Co	?	+
Ni	?	+
As	0	?
Se	0	+
Sn	0	?
I	0	+

† Key: +, generally required; 0, not established as generally required; ?, evidence for general essentiality not yet conclusive.

‡ Sodium is considered a micronutrient for plant species having the C_4 dicarboxylic acid photosynthetic pathway. It is a macronutrient for animals.

Knowledge concerning the movement of many mineral elements through the food chain is meager. Almost nothing is known about either the available levels of the newer essential trace elements in soils, factors that influence their concentration in edible plant parts, or the influence of various dietary and environmental factors on their bioavailability to animals and humans.

Various human activities may result in marginal deficiencies or toxicities of certain trace mineral elements in plants, animals, and people (Allaway, 1968; Kubota et al., 1977; Lepp, 1981; Lisk, 1972; Underwood, 1979a, 1979b, 1979c). Examples of these activities and some concerns generated by them are listed in Table 2.

Several recent developments have greatly increased the awareness of nutritionists to potential mineral nutrient deficiencies in humans (Mertz, 1981b; Underwood, 1977, 1979c, 1981). One was the discovery of Zn deficiency in people in developing countries, and subsequently in developed countries (Hambidge, 1981). Endemic Se deficiencies in people of the Keshan region of China were revealed recently (Zhu, 1981). The widespread occurrence of Fe-deficiency anemia in people, as reported in nutritional surveys conducted in Canada and the United States (Abraham et al., 1974; Sabry et al., 1974), also has served to stimulate interest in mineral nutrients. Finally, the recent report that inadequate Ca intake may be a previously unrecognized causal factor in hypertension in humans has given further impetus to increased interest in mineral nutrition, especially in light of the fact that Ca intake is decreasing in the United States (McCarron et al., 1982).

Table 2. Examples of some human activities which may result in marginal deficiency or toxicity of certain mineral elements for plants, animals, and people.

Activity	Concern
1. Use of contaminated sewage sludge, fly ash, and waste products on agricultural land.	1. Excessive plant levels of Cd, Hg, and other metal antagonists of mineral bioavailability.
2. Decreased use of Cu fungicides.	2. Decreased Cu levels in edible plants.
3. Increased use of excessive P fertilizers on marginally Zn-deficient lands.	3. Decreased Zn levels in edible plants.
4. Decreased use of galvanized plumbing for water supplies.	4. Decreased Zn levels in potable water.
5. Changes in source of raw materials for use in commercial fertilizer production.	5. Increases in toxic heavy metals (e.g., Cd) or decreases in essential trace elements (Zn).
6. Increases in chemical purity of commercially available fertilizers	6. Loss of essential trace element impurities (e.g., Zn, Cu, and Mn).
7. Increased consumption of highly refined plant food products.	7. Decreased intake of certain essential trace elements (e.g., Zn).
8. Decreased availability and consumption of a wide variety of food sources	8. Decreased probability of consuming adequate levels of essential mineral nutrients.
9. Increased consumption of plant foods replacing animal protein in human diets.	9. Decreased bioavailability of essential trace metals (e.g., Fe and Zn) and Ca in human diets.
10. Breeding of high-yielding varieties of crops for total yield or protein quality.	10. Little attention given to mineral nutrient content of new varieties.

Summarizing, there is increasing concern about the concentration and bioavailability of mineral nutrients in plant foods. Increased awareness of mineral nutritional problems in humans has increased the need to evaluate the role of different food crops in supplying humans with adequate, available levels of these nutrients. The naturally occurring levels, or so-called "background" levels, of many different essential and toxic trace elements, along with the important environmental factors that influence their levels, in food crops need to be studied in greater detail (Kubota and Allaway, 1972). These studies must be bolstered by an evaluation of mineral bioavailability to people and of those factors in plant foods that affect it. Armed with this knowledge, scientists can make rational decisions concerning whether or not to increase essential element levels in food crops up to a level sufficient to meet human requirements. If current agronomic practices, such as fertilization and crop breeding programs, cannot be used economically to improve mineral composition and increase the bioavailability of mineral nutrients in food crops, then direct dietary supplementation of the limiting nutrients may be desirable. However, even if this latter option is chosen, to supplement diets effectively, the range of essential element levels and their bioavailability (and factors that affect it) in human food crops must be known and understood.

BIOAVAILABILITY IN RELATION TO RECOMMENDED DIETARY ALLOWANCES

Recommended Dietary Allowances (RDA) are defined as "estimates of the amounts of essential nutrients each person in a healthy population must consume in order to provide reasonable assurance that the physio-

Table 3. Information required to establish realistic recommended dietary allowances.

1. Metabolic needs.
2. Variability among individuals.
3. Changes in requirement with changes in physiological state.
4. Reliable analytical methods for determining nutrient composition of food.
5. Reasonable degree of accuracy in determining nutrient bioavailability and factors that affect it.

Table 4. Examples of suggested promoters or inhibitors of mineral nutrient bioavailability in various plant foods.

Component	Some elements affected	Examples of plant foods
Potential inhibitors		
Fibrous carbohydrates	Zn	Whole cereal grains
Goitrogens	I	Species of *Brassica* (e.g., cabbage), soybeans
High Cd	Fe, Zn, Cu, Se, Ca	Contaminated leafy vegetables and rice grain
High Mo	Cu	Sorghum high in Mo
Long chain fatty acids	Ca, Mg	Possibly oil seeds
Oxalic acid	Ca	Oxalate accumulators (e.g., spinach)
Phytic acid	Zn	Mature seeds and whole cereal grains
Tannins (polyphenolics)	Fe	Coffee, Tea
Potential promoters		
Ascorbic acid	Fe	Citrus fruits
Vitamin D	Ca, P	No edible plants are known to be high in vitamin D

logical needs of all will be met". Some define them simply as "safe acceptable nutrient intakes" (Harper, 1976). Various factors must be considered when determining RDA's (Harper, 1976; National Research Council, 1980). Some of these are listed in Table 3. Despite concern over the capability of some diets to meet certain micronutrient requirements of humans, only 3 of 15 essential trace elements (Fe, Zn, and I) are included in the table of dietary allowances.

Estimating the bioavailability to humans of mineral nutrients in complex diets is one of the major problems encountered in formulating an accurate mineral nutrient RDA (Harper, 1976). Plant foods are of special concern because they may contain factors which either promote or diminish the bioavailability to humans of some mineral nutrients (Davies, 1979; Gontzea and Sutzescu, 1968). A number of these components are shown in Table 4. It should be stressed that many of the inhibitors and promoters listed are still very controversial factors; much more research is required before conclusive proof of their negative or positive role in mineral nutrient bioavailability is obtained.

The difficulties encountered in calculating required mineral nutrient levels in human diets are substantial. The method used to calculate available Fe levels in meals provides a good example of some of the complexities faced when one determines whether or not certain meals contain adequate amounts of mineral nutrients (National Research Council, 1980). In the United States, five variables are presently recommended for calculating absorbable Fe in human diets. These include the content of total Fe, heme Fe, nonheme Fe, ascorbic acid, and animal tissues in the

Table 5. Categories of meal types currently used in the United States
for evaluating Fe availability in different meals. †

Meal types	Percentage Fe absorbed from meal	
	Nonheme Fe	Heme Fe
Low Fe availability	3	23
< 30 g animal tissues		
< 25 mg ascorbic acid		
Medium Fe availability	5	23
30–90 g animal tissue		
or 25–75 mg ascorbic acid		
High Fe availability	8	23
> 90 g animal tissues		
or > 75 mg ascorbic acid		
or 30–90 g animal tissues		
plus 25–75 mg ascorbic acid		

† Adapted from National Research Council, 1980.

meal. Amounts of total Fe and ascorbic acid in food are obtained from values listed in standard food composition tables. Nonheme Fe is calculated by subtracting heme Fe (assumed to be 40% of total Fe in animal tissues) from total Fe. Using these values, meals are classified into three categories as shown in Table 5 (National Research Council, 1980). Both the amounts of animal tissue and ascorbic acid are included in these calculations because both are known to be factors that can strongly affect the amount of Fe absorbed. Heme Fe is absorbed from the intestine by a different mechanism than nonheme Fe. Heme and nonheme Fe are thought to occur as independent, nonexchangeable Fe pools in the alimentary tract. Estimates are that about 23% of the heme Fe is absorbed from a meal. Nonheme Fe absorption can vary greatly depending on a number of factors including the level of ascorbic acid (a strong promoter of nonheme Fe absorption under certain circumstances) in the meal (Mertz, 1980; National Research Council, 1980).

The absorption values listed in Table 5 are applicable only to individuals who are not Fe deficient. Because of homeostatic mechanisms controlling Fe absorption in the human body, actual absorption percentages can be substantially higher for Fe deficient people. Iron-depleted individuals absorb Fe more efficiently than Fe-adequate people (Underwood, 1977). Individuals with very high body stores of Fe may have much lower absorption percentages than listed in Table 5. Iron-adequate individuals absorb less Fe because they require less to maintain Fe balance (Underwood, 1977).

Currently it is commonly thought that many important food crops, such as edible legume seeds and cereal grains which lack significant amounts of heme Fe or ascorbic acid, are poor sources of available Fe. However, not all research supports this conclusion (see references cited in Bothwell et al., 1982; Morris and Ellis, 1980; Welch and Van Campen, 1975; Young and Janghorbani, 1981). Research is needed to determine whether or not these plant foods are poor sources of available Fe and, if so, what are the causal factors.

Table 6. Methods commonly used to determine bioavailability of mineral nutrients in foods.

1. Chemical balance studies
   a. percent apparent digestibility
   b. percent apparent retention
2. Isotope methods (radioisotopes and stable isotopes)
   a. index of availability
   b. true absorption
   c. whole-body retention
   d. true digestibility
   e. isotope balance
3. Relative biological values

The example of Fe has shown the importance of bioavailability in determining appropriate RDAs. Present estimates of the bioavailability of many essential mineral nutrients in plant foods may be either too high or too low. The bioavailability of the newer essential trace elements has not been determined for most food crops. Without accurate estimates of the amount of available mineral nutrients in edible plants, realistic RDA's cannot be determined.

FACTORS AFFECTING MINERAL NUTRIENT BIOAVAILABILITY

One of the most serious problems facing nutritionists interested in the bioavailability of mineral nutrients is methodology. The reported values for the bioavailability of many essential minerals in human diets varies greatly depending on the method used to determine them. There are no reliable standard methods presently available whereby the values reported by different laboratories can be compared directly. Numerous methods currently in use include various types of chemical balance trials, isotopic tracer procedures and relative biological value procedures (see Table 6). None of these methods are without problems (Janghorbani and Young, 1980a; Lengemann, 1974). New methods using stable isotopes of mineral nutrients are currently under development in several laboratories and they may help to clarify the confusion that exists in the nutrition literature regarding the bioavailability of mineral nutrients in food crops and factors that affect them (Janghorbani and Young, 1980a, 1980b; Johnson, 1982; Miller and Van Campen, 1979; Turnlund et al., 1982).

Table 7 lists selected factors considered to affect the bioavailability of several mineral nutrients in plant foods. Table 8 lists some of these factors in a different format stressing their interrelationships. These consumer, dietary, and environmental factors all interact and much remains to be learned about how they interact to affect specific mineral nutrients.

Several compounds that occur naturally in edible plants are considered to be antinutritive substances (Table 4). Some of these compounds may be responsible for the low bioavailability of certain mineral nutrients in plant foods (Davis, 1979; Gontzea and Sutzescu, 1968; Liener, 1980; Underwood, 1977; Widdowson, 1980). For example, oxalic acid has been reported to be an antinutrient. Certain plants, such as rhubarb (*Rheum*

Table 7. Examples of factors affecting mineral nutrient bioavailability.

1. Chemical form of the element in the diet
2. Interactions with other elements at sites of:
     a. absorption
     b. storage
     c. utilization
     d. excretion
3. Interactions with organic compounds of diets:
     a. protein (e.g., plant vs. animal)
     b. amino acids (e.g., arginine, histidine, cysteine)
     c. organic acids (e.g., ascorbic acid, citric acid, phytic acid, oxalic acid, long chain fatty acids)
     d. carbohydrates
          1. fibrous (e.g., cellulose, hemicellulose, pectin)
          2. sugars (e.g., fructose, lactose)
     e. tannins (e.g., polyphenols)
4. Physiological state of individual
     a. tissue stores
     b. genetic variables
     c. diseases
          1. malabsorption disorders
          2. pathogens
          3. parasites
     d. anabolic demands (e.g., growth rate, age, pregnancy, lactation)
     e. trauma and stress
     f. physicochemical condition of digesta in alimentary tract

Table 8. Interactions of factors affecting the value of plant foods as sources of essential mineral nutrients for humans.

Consumer Factors	Dietary Factors	Environmental Factors
Physiological status	Amount of element in diet	Geographical location and soil type
Nutritional status	Chemical form of element	Postharvest handling and storage
Hereditary factors	Nutritive promoters	Plant species and varieties
Economic status	Dietary composition	Processing and preparation
Disease status	Antinutritives	Management practices
	Element interactions	Plant age and part eaten
		Climate

rhaponticum L.) and spinach (*Spinacia oleracea* L.) accumulate rather high levels of oxalic acid. Because oxalate forms insoluble precipitates with Ca ions, it has been shown to reduce the bioavailability of Ca if ingested in high concentrations under certain circumstances (Gontzea and Sutzescu, 1968). However, in a critical evaluation of the consumption of oxalate accumulator plants by people, it was concluded that there is very little danger associated with the eating of these plants. For oxalate to have a detrimental effect, a very high intake of the oxalate accumulating plants would have to occur simultaneously with a very low intake of both Ca and vitamin D over a long period of time (Liener, 1980). In relation to other cations, recent reports do not substantiate the dogma that oxalate reduces either Fe or Zn bioavailability (Van Campen and Welch, 1980; Welch et al., 1977). Apparently, the influence of oxalate on multivalent cation nutrient bioavailability is neither a significant nor a common nutritional problem.

Various antinutritional properties have been attributed to phytic acid (myo-inositolhexaphosphoric acid), the major storage form of P in mature seeds. This compound has been reported to be responsible for the low availability to humans and animals of Fe, Zn, Ca, and other multivalent cations in mature seeds and grains (Gontzea and Sutzescu, 1968; Oberleas, 1973). Phytic acid forms insoluble precipitates in vitro with various multivalent cations at pH's similar to those measured inside the lumen of the small intestine (i.e., greater than pH 7) (Byrd and Matrone, 1965; Vohra et al., 1965). One proposed mechanism of action in vivo is the formation of insoluble coprecipitates of Ca phytate with other polyvalent cations, possibly in conjunction with mixed precipitates of certain types of protein found in seeds (O'Dell, 1969). The formation of these insoluble precipitates was thought to be responsible for the decreased absorption of these cations. This argument was used to explain the low bioavailability of these nutrients to monogastric animals fed meals containing mature seeds and grains. However, the presence of high levels of naturally occurring phytic acid salts (i.e., phytin) in complex diets does not always substantially depress the bioavailability of many multivalent cations. In fact, monoferric-phytate, a soluble form of Fe reported to occur naturally in cereal grains, is apparently a good source of available Fe to monogastric animals (Morris and Ellis, 1976). Additionally, the level of phytin in diets cannot always be used to predict the bioavailability of other polyvalent cations. Other unknown factors (e.g., fiber) may also be involved.

The major chemical forms of mineral nutrients in edible plant tissues may also play an important role in mineral nutrient bioavailability (Davies, 1979; Quarterman, 1973). Unfortunately, very little is known about the naturally occurring forms of most mineral nutrients. A few have been identified (e.g., monoferric phytate in wheat grain; Morris and Ellis, 1976); some have been reported to be small molecular weight soluble anionic metal complexes, but their identification has been elusive (Tinker, 1981; Walker and Welch, 1981). Without knowledge of their identity, experiments to determine their direct effects on bioavailability cannot be performed. Some of these compounds may be either promoters or inhibitors of mineral nutrient bioavailability. Because some of these compounds do form very stable complexes with some cations such as Zn, they may prevent the precipitation of these multivalent cations by phytin or other antinutritives in the intestinal lumen. Research should be intensified to characterize and identify these compounds in food crops.

The activity of the endogenous intestinal enzyme phytase (an alkaline phosphatase which hydrolyzes phosphate groups from phytic acid) illustrates another complicating factor which may play an important role in determining the amount of phytin required to decrease the bioavailability of multivalent cations. Hydrolysis of phytin by this enzyme would destroy the molecule's ability to precipitate cations. Some evidence (D. R. Van Campen, personal communication) suggests that phytase may be inhibited by high levels of the substrate it hydrolyzes (i.e., phytic acid). Therefore, continuous ingestion of meals high in phytin might result in diminished bioavailability of cations as a result of phytin inhibition of phytase. Thus, hypothetically, western style diets may be less at risk in regards to the negative effects of phytin than are some diets

Table 9. Areas of research where expanded effort should provide the knowledge needed to improve the bioavailability of mineral nutrients in plant foods.

1. Identification of major forms and levels of essential elements in edible plant products.
2. Identification, level, interactions, and mode of action of both antinutritive and promoter factors in edible plant products which affect essential element bioavailability.
3. Understanding of the basic mechanisms of absorption of essential mineral nutrients in the human alimentary tract.
4. Reliable, convenient, standard methods for determining mineral nutrient bioavailability in human subjects or the development of reliable animals models and/or in vitro assays.

in developing countries, because they normally do not include the continuous ingestion of high phytin meals primarily composed of foods prepared from whole grains or mature seeds.

These examples point out some of the difficulties encountered when studying mineral inhibitor and promoter factors in human diets. Clearly, the diversity of foods in various meals and the complexities of the human digestive system do not lend themselves to simplistic views of the bioavailability of most mineral nutrients in human diets. A great deal of research is still required before scientists can accurately predict the bioavailability of mineral nutrients in plant foods. Table 9 gives some examples of the types of research needed to attain this goal.

AGRONOMIC PRACTICES AND THE MINERAL NUTRIENT QUALITY OF CROPS

What agronomic practices can be employed to improve food crops as sources of essential elements? The transfer of essential nutrient elements from soils to plants and ultimately into human diets is a very complicated process. Many interrelated factors, both genetic and environmental, control their movement. Each element, as it traverses the food chain, may follow its own unique route which may be regulated by specific mechanisms. Thus, broad generalizations covering all mineral nutrients are risky. Therefore, to answer the question posed, one is forced to evaluate specific mineral nutrients, in specific food crops, grown in similar environments (Allaway, 1968, 1975).

Availability to plants of mineral nutrients in soils can be influenced by various soil management factors. Some of these factors are drainage, acidity, organic matter content, cultivation, and the application of chemical fertilizers (Allaway, 1968; West, 1981). Poor drainage and resulting reducing conditions can greatly increase the availability of some essential trace elements in soils to plants. However, impeded drainage is not a viable soil management practice because it normally causes severe problems for plant growth. Likewise, lowering the acidity of a soil by such practices as adding lime can greatly affect the availability of many essential trace elements to plants (e.g., lowering available Fe, Zn, Mn, and Ni and increasing available Mo and Se). Here, too, the beneficial effects of lime on plant growth outweighs its detrimental effects of reducing certain trace element concentrations in plants. Similarly, the addition of organic matter to soils generally has a beneficial effect on various soil properties, including increased availability of some essential trace elements (Allaway, 1968; West, 1981). However, organic matter is not a panacea for improving the essential nutrient content of food crops (Allaway, 1975; Beeson and Matrone, 1976). The mineral nutrient content of different sources of organic matter varies greatly depending on the type of organic material and its origin. Some organic matter derived from plant materials grown on soils low in various essential trace elements (e.g., I and Co) contain very low levels of these elements and cannot be used to increase the available level of these nutrients to growing plants. Cultivation of soils by man can also have a significant effect on availability of some mineral nutrients to plants (West, 1981). Conventional plowing practices mix surface soil horizons and tend to uniformly distribute mineral nutrients in the rooting zone of plants. Minimum tillage may affect mineral nutrient availability to plants, but the effects of minimum tillage on mineral availability remains to be determined. The consequences of soil compaction resulting from the ever increasing size and weight of farm machinery can also have an effect on the mineral composition of crops. For example, the concentrations of Ca, K, Mg, and Mn in pea (*Pisum sativum* L.) shoots were reduced by application of mechanical stress to soils (Castillo et al., 1982). These reductions were related to restricted root distribution in the soil. Other nutrients studied (i.e., B, Fe, and P) were not affected by mechanical stress. Compressing soil around roots during tillage operations may reduce root length and nutrient uptake much more than that resulting from plants grown in more compacted soils under reduced tillage systems. Manipulating soil tillage practices, however, cannot increase the available mineral nutrient content of soils with inadequate stores of nutrients. Thus, of the soil management practices listed, the use of chemical fertilizers has the greatest potential to raise the level of specific mineral nutrients in food crops grown on soils having specific nutrient deficiencies.

The use of macronutrient fertilizers (e.g., N, P, and K) may result in changes in the concentration of nutritionally important minerals and in certain antinutritive compounds, in edible plants (Allaway, 1968, 1971, 1975; Peck et al., 1980; West, 1981). For example, the use of P fertilizers, while improving yields, may depress trace element concentrations in plants (see Fig. 1) and increase the concentration of phytic acid (see Table 10). The depressing effect of macronutrient fertilizers on lowering trace element levels in plants is not a universal phenomenon because there are instances where excessive levels of P have increased levels of trace elements in plant tissues (West, 1981). Further, trace element impurities in some commercial fertilizers and soil amendments can slightly increase the level of available trace elements in soils (Lisk, 1972). Very little is known about the effects of macronutrient fertilizers on trace element availability to plants. Thus far, only a minor influence has been observed within the range of normal fertilization practices (West, 1981).

The use of specific fertilizers to increase the essential element content of food crops can be effective for some mineral elements but has not been a successful practice for others. Most plants appear to have certain mechanisms for controlling the level of some nutrients in their tissues and

Table 10. Effect of P fertilizer on phytic acid concentration in immature and mature pea seeds. †

	Phytic acid	
Phosphorus fertilizer	Immature seeds	Mature seeds
kg ha⁻¹	mol kg⁻¹ dry wt	
0	0.11	0.27
30	0.13	0.30
60	0.14	0.33
120	0.15	0.35

† Peck et al., 1980.

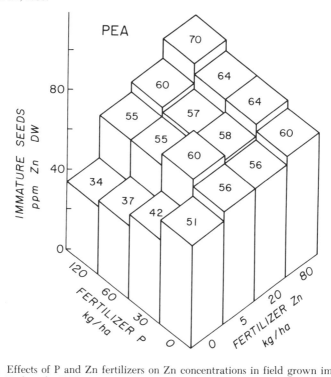

Fig. 1. Effects of P and Zn fertilizers on Zn concentrations in field grown immature pea seeds (Peck et al., 1980).

normally do not concentrate these nutrients beyond a certain level even if supplied in excessive but nontoxic amounts (Clarkson and Hanson, 1980). For example, it has not been possible to substantially increase the Fe, Mn, Ca, or V content of edible portions of food crops by excessive fertilization with soluble compounds of these elements (Allaway, 1971; Beeson and Matrone, 1976; National Research Council, 1974, 1977). However, for other essential elements, such as Zn, fertilization with available forms of these elements, under some circumstances, may substantially increase mineral concentrations in edible plant tissues (Peck et al., 1980; Welch et al., 1974; Welch and House, 1982). On some soils that have inadequate levels of both available P and Zn, heavy applications of P fertilizers can increase the severity of Zn deficiency symptoms in many crops (Olsen,

Table 11. Effect of increasing Zn supply in nutrient solution on Zn concentration, Zn bioavailability, and percentage of RDA on Zn supplied by 100 g of pea seeds. [†]

Zinc in nutrient solution	Growth stage	Zinc concentration in seed (dry wt.)	Zinc bioavail- ability	Percent of Zn RDA met per 100 g of seeds[‡]
		μmol kg^{-1}		%
Low	Immature (green)	337	95	14
(1 μmol L^{-1})	Mature	138	77	5
High	Immature (green)	765	90	30
(4 μmol L^{-1})	Mature	719	75	24

[†] Welch et al., 1974.
[‡] RDA for mature men and women is 15 mg of Zn per day.

1972). Not only are crop yields depressed by Zn deficiency but also the concentration of Zn in the edible plant tissues can be decreased. The data shown in Fig. 1 demonstrate this point. Thus, the nutritional value of these crops with respect to Zn is diminished. Under these circumstances concomitant P and Zn fertilization can give nutritionally beneficial results (Peck et al., 1980). As expected, yields improve and also, as seen in Fig. 1, the concentration of Zn in edible plant parts increases greatly.

Whether or not increased Zn in plant tissues, that results from Zn fertilization, is available for absorption by monogastric animals has been tested using immature and mature pea seeds (Welch et al., 1974) and soybeans [*Glycine max* (L.) Merr.] (Welch and House, 1982) fed to rats. Table 11 shows that the bioavailability of Zn in pea seeds is not reduced by Zn fertilization. The percent of the Zn RDA from 100 g of mature pea seeds was increased almost fivefold by increasing the Zn supplied to the pea plant. Thus, fertilization with available forms of Zn can result in improvements in nutritional quality of some food crops. Possibly, Zn fertilization rates, in excess of those required for maximum yield may be desirable.

Selection of more nutritious plant strains through plant breeding practices is another means by which food crops may be improved as sources of available mineral nutrients for humans. Two approaches could be used in the selection process. One is to breed for plant genotypes that accumulate greater amounts of specific mineral nutrients in edible plant parts. Another is to select genotypes of food crops that contain fewer inhibitors or more promoters of mineral nutrient bioavailability. Hypothetically, the latter approach could produce undesirable consequences for plant growth and productivity. For example, if one bred for a genotype that accumulated less phytin in its seeds, lower P stores would be accumulated in the seeds. This could result in decreased resistance in the seed to phosphate deficiency stress and in depressed seed vigor. Seeds containing low phytin levels would have less chance of survival when germinated in soils low in available P, or the seedlings produced from these seeds could have slower growth rates than normal seedlings when grown under these conditions. Therefore, caution should be exercised when trying to decrease the level of compounds in plant foods that inhibit mineral nutrient bioavailability.

Another drawback to the second approach is the lack of adequate knowledge concerning the identity of inhibitors or promoters of mineral nutrient bioavailability in plant foods. Presently, it is not possible to advise plant breeders as to which compounds are responsible for reduced bioavailability of various essential mineral elements in plant foods. Many proposed inhibitor compounds have been suggested, but none have been conclusively shown to be responsible for the observed reductions in bioavailability of mineral nutrients. The same holds for promoters of mineral nutrient bioavailability. Many naturally occurring compounds have been proposed, but only a few have been shown to be effective (e.g., ascorbic acid in promoting Fe availability). Thus, this approach awaits much more research before it is a viable alternative for plant breeders.

Therefore, plant breeders are currently left with the first alternative; that is, selecting for genotypes that accumulate specific mineral nutrients in edible portions of crops. Differences between crops for selective uptake and utilization of mineral nutrients are known (Brown et al., 1972; Epstein, 1972). Plant breeders are studying the differences between plant efficiencies in the use of mineral elements in order to increase the adaptation of crops to mineral stresses in problem soils (Graham, 1983; Wright and Ferrari, 1976). Knowledge gained through this type of research could be used to improve food crops as sources of mineral nutrients. Presently, selecting food crops bred for accumulating specific mineral nutrients in edible plant parts, in conjunction with fertilization practices to increase available supplies of those nutrients in soils, would appear to be the most worthwhile approach to use in improving crops as sources of mineral nutrients for humans.

RESEARCH FOR THE FUTURE

Ca, Fe, and Zn are some mineral nutrients which may be limiting in diets of some population groups worldwide. Also, Mg, Cu, Cr, Se, and other newer essential trace elements are presently of growing concern to human nutritionists. Thus, any research directed at increasing the available levels of these nutrients in food crops could make important improvements in the nutritional health of people.

About one-third (on a dry weight basis) of the food consumed in the United States is comprised of plant products of mature seed or grain origin (U.S. Department of Agriculture, 1981). Thus, edible seeds and gains are a major source of some essential mineral nutrients for people in this country. In the future, more dependence will be placed on these plant foods if per capita consumption of animal tissues decline. In general, plant seeds and grains lack adequate available quantities of several essential minerals (e.g., Ca, Zn, and Fe) and do not provide the RDAs of these nutrients. Most past research has been directed at increasing crop yields. Very little has been done on improving the mineral nutrient quality of food crops and most of this research has dealt with edible plant roots and leaves. As a result, very little is known about the mechanisms

Table 12. Examples of soil-root interface processes where lack of sufficient knowledge is hindering progress towards improved mineral nutrient quality of crops.

1. Chemical and biological processes in soils which control the solubility of mineral nutrients in soil solution.
2. Physical, chemical, and biological processes limiting the movement of essential mineral elements to root surfaces.
3. Basic mechanisms controlling the absorption of mineral nutrients by roots (especially micronutrients and trace elements).
4. Processes controlling interactions between mineral nutrients and other elements in the soil-plant system.

controlling the mobilization, translocation, and deposition of essential minerals in plant seeds and grains. Lack of such knowledge has prevented the development of practices which could be used to increase the level of nutritionally important essential metals in edible seeds and grains. Thus, much more research on the physiology of plants is needed to develop an understanding of the mechanisms whereby essential mineral nutrients are deposited in edible seeds and grains. Without this research, dramatic improvements in the mineral nutritional quality of seeds and grains will be difficult.

Limited knowledge in other areas of soil-plant interactions is also slowing the development of food crops having greater mineral nutrient quality. Some examples of research areas within the soil-root interface system are listed in Table 12. Increased research effort in these areas could hasten improvements in crop quality.

SUMMARY

Plant foods are important sources of mineral nutrients for humans. Thus, the bioavailability of essential elements in edible plant products is an important consideration when establishing realistic RDAs. Yet, because of: (1) the unknown nature of the major chemical forms of mineral nutrients in plant foods; (2) the presence of various antinutritive factors and promoters of mineral nutrient absorption in plant products which affect mineral nutrient absorption and utilization; (3) the complexity and diversity of varied human diets; (4) the complexity and the incomplete and rudimentary understanding of mineral absorption processes in the alimentary tract; and (5) the inherent difficulties of research using human subjects, only empirical estimates of bioavailability of mineral nutrients in plant foods are presently available for use in calculating RDAs. Much basic research is still required on those factors in plant foods which inhibit or facilitate mineral nutrient absorption before accurate estimates of the bioavailability of essential elements can be made. Without more basic knowledge of how plant constituents, mineral nutrients, and absorption mechanisms in humans interact, progress will be slow to develop more nutritious plant foods through either plant breeding programs or agronomic practices.

REFERENCES

1. Abraham, S., F. W. Lowenstein, and C. L. Johnson. 1974. Preliminary findings of the first health and nutrition examination survey, United States, 1971–1972. Department of Health, Education and Welfare Publ. No. (HRA) 74-1219-1, Washington, D.C.

2. Allaway, W. H. 1968. Agronomic controls over the environmental cycling of trace elements. Adv. Agron. 20:235–274.

3. ————. 1971. Feed and food quality in relation to fertilizer use. p. 533–555. *In* Fertilizer technology and use. Soil Sci. Soc. of Am., Madison, Wis.

4. ————. 1975. The effect of soils and fertilizers on human and animal nutrition. USDA Agric. Inform. Bull. 378.

5. Ammerman, C. B., and S. M. Miller. 1972. Biological availability of minor mineral ions: a review. J. Anim. Sci. 35:681–694.

6. Beeson, K. C., A. L. Forbes, D. J. Horvath, and F. W. Lowenstein. 1978. Plants and foods of plant origin. p. 59–78. *In* Geochemistry and the environment, Vol. III. Natl. Acad. Sci., Washington, D.C.

7. ————, and G. Matrone. 1976. The soil factor in nutrition. Marcel Dekker, Inc., New York.

8. Bothwell, T. H., F. M. Clydesdale, J. D. Cook, P. R. Dallman, L. Hallberg, D. Van Campen, and W. Wolf. 1982. The effects of cereals and legumes on iron availability. Internatl. Nutr. Anemia Consultative Group. The Nutr. Foundation, Washington, D.C.

9. Bremner, I., and C. F. Mills. 1981. Absorption, transport, and tissue storage of essential trace elements. Phil. Trans. R. Soc. Lond. B294:75–89.

10. Brown, J.C., J. E. Ambler, R. L. Chaney, and C. D.Foy. 1972. Differential responses of plant genotypes to micronutrients. p. 389–418. *In* J. M. Mortvedt, P. M. Giordano, and W. L. Lindsay (ed.) Micronutrients in agriculture. Soil Sci. Soc. of Am., Madison, Wis.

11. Byrd, C. A., and G. Matrone. 1965. Investigations of chemical basis of zinc-calcium-phytate interaction in biological systems. Soc. Exp. Biol. Med. 119:347–349.

12. Castillo, S. R., R. H. Dowdy, J. M. Bradford, and W. E. Larson. 1982. Effects of applied mechanical stress on plant growth and nutrient uptake. Agron. J. 74:526–530.

13. Chesters, J. K. 1976. Trace elements: adventitious yet essential dietary ingredients. Proc. Nutr. Soc. 35:15–22.

14. Clarkson, D. T., and J. B. Hanson. 1980. The mineral nutrition of plants. Ann. Rev. Plant Physiol. 31:239–298.

15. Davies, N. T. 1979. Anti-nutrient factors affecting mineral utilization. Proc. Nutr. Soc. 38:121–128.

16. Epstein, E. 1972. Mineral nutrition of plants: principles and perspectives. John Wiley and Sons, Inc., New York.

17. Fritz, J. C. 1973. Effect of processing on the availability and nutritional value of trace mineral elements. p. 109–118. *In* Effect of processing on the nutritional value of feeds. Natl. Acad. Sci., Washington, D.C.

18. Gontzea, I., and P. Sutzescu. 1968. Natural antinutritive substances in foodstuffs and forages. S. Karger, Basel, Switzerland.

19. Goodhart, R. S., and M. E. Shils. 1980. Modern nutrition in health and disease. Lea and Febiger, Philadelphia, Penn.

20. Graham, R. D. 1984. Breeding for nutritional characteristics in cereals. Adv. Plant Nutr. 1:(In press).

21. Hambidge, K. M. 1981. Zinc deficiency in man: its origins and effects. Phil. Trans. R. Soc. Lond. B294:129–144.

22. Harper, A. E. 1976. Basis of recommended dietary allowances for trace elements. p. 371–378. *In* A. S. Prasad and D. Oberleas (ed.) Trace elements in human health and disease. Academic Press, Inc., New York.

23. Janghorbani, M., and V. R. Young. 1980a. Stable isotope methods for bioavailability assessment of dietary minerals in humans. p. 127–155. In H. H. Draper (ed.) Advances in nutritional research, Vol. 3. Plenum Press, New York.

24. ----, and ----. 1980b. Use of stable isotopes to determine bioavailability of minerals in human diets using the method of fecal monitoring. Am. J. Clin. Nutr. 33:2021–2030.

25. Johnson, P. E. 1982. A mass spectrometric method for use of stable isotopes as tracers in studies of iron, zinc, and copper absorption in human subjects. J. Nutr. 112:1414–1424.

26. Kubota, J., and W. H. Allaway. 1972. Geographic distribution of trace element problems. p. 525–554. In J. J. Mortvedt, P. M. Giordano, and W. L. Lindsay (ed.) Micronutrients in agriculture. Soil Sci. Soc. of Am., Madison, Wis.

27. ----, K. C. Beeson, T. D. Hinesly, E. A. Jenne, W. L. Lindsay, and P. R. Stout. 1977. Consequences of soil imbalances. p. 116–119. In Geochemistry and the environment, Vol. II. Natl. Acad. Sci., Washington, D.C.

28. Lengemann, F. W. 1974. Mineral and trace mineral disease studies with tracers. p. 47–60. In Tracer techniques in tropical animal production. Internatl. Atomic Energy Agency, Vienna, Austria.

29. Lepp, N. W. (ed.) 1981. Effect of heavy metal pollution on plants, Vol. 2. Applied Science Publishers Ltd., London.

30. Liener, I. E. 1980. Miscellaneous toxic factors. p. 429–467. In I. E. Liener (ed.) Toxic constituents of plant foodstuffs. Academic Press, Inc., New York.

31. Lisk, D. J. 1972. Trace metals in soils, plants, and animals. Adv. Agron. 24:267–325.

32. McCarron, D. A., C. D. Morris, and C. Cole. 1982. Dietary calcium in human hypertension. Sci. 217:267–269.

33. Mertz, W. 1980. Trace mineral elements, mammalian requirements and man's presumptive needs. p. 257–271. In K. Blaxter (ed.) Food chains and human nutrition. Applied Science Publishers Ltd., London.

34. Mertz, W. 1981a. The essential trace elements. Sci. 213:1332–1338.

35. ----. 1981b. The scientific and practical importance of trace elements. Phil. Trans. R. Soc. Lond. B294:9–18.

36. Miller, D. D., and D. Van Campen. 1979. A method for the detection and assay of iron stable isotope tracers in blood serum. Am. J. Clin. Nutr. 32:2354–2361.

37. Morris, E. R., and R. Ellis. 1976. Isolation of monoferric phytate from wheat bran and its biological value as an iron source to the rat. J. Nutr. 106:753–760.

38. ----, and ----. 1980. Bioavailability to rats of iron and zinc in wheat bran: response to low-phytate bran and effect of the phytate/zinc molar ratio. J. Nutr. 110:2000–2010.

39. National Research Council. 1974. Geochemistry and the environment, Vol. I. The relation of selected trace elements to health and disease. Natl. Acad. Sci., Washington, D.C.

40. ----. 1977. Geochemistry and the environment, Vol. II. The relation of other selected trace elements to health and disease. Natl. Acad. Sci., Washington, D.C.

41. ----, Committee on Dietary Allowances, Food and Nutrition Board. 1980. Recommended dietary allowances. Natl. Acad. Sci., Washington, D.C.

42. Oberleas, D. 1973. Phytates. p. 363–371. In Toxicants occurring naturally in foods. Natl. Acad. Sci., Washington, D.C.

43. O'Dell, B. L. 1969. Effect of dietary components upon zinc availability: a review with original data. Am. J. Clin. Nutr. 10:1315–1322.

44. Olsen, S. R. 1972. Micronutrient interactions. p. 243–264. In J. M. Mortvedt, P. M. Giordano, and W. L. Lindsay (ed.) Micronutrients in agriculture. Soil Sci. Soc. of Am., Madison, Wis.

45. Peck, N. H., D. L. Grunes, R. M. Welch, and G. E. MacDonald. 1980. Nutritional quality of vegetable crops as affected by P and zinc fertilizers. Agron. J. 72:528–534.

46. Quarterman, J. 1973. Factors which influence the amount and availability of trace elements in human food plants. Qual. Plant. Plant Foods Hum. Nutr. 23:171–190.

47. Sabry, Z. I., J. A. Campbell, M. E. Campbell, and A. L. Forbes. 1974. Nutrition Canada. Nutr. Today 9:5–13.

48. Tinker, P. B. 1981. Levels, distribution and chemical forms of trace elements in food plants. Phil. Trans. R. Soc. Lond. B294:41–55.

49. Turnlund, J. R., M. C. Michel, W. R. Keyes, J. C. King, and S. Margen. 1982. Use of enriched stable isotopes to determine zinc and iron absorption in elderly men. Am. J. Clin. Nutr. 35:1033–1040.

50. Underwood, E. J. 1977. Trace elements in human and animal nutrition. Academic Press, New York.

51. ––––. 1979a. Trace elements and health: an overview. Phil. Trans. R. Soc. Lond. B288: 5–14.

52. ––––. 1979b. Environmental sources of heavy metals and their toxicity to man and animals. Prog. Water Tech. 11:33–45.

53. ––––. 1979c. Trace metals in human and animal health. J. Roy. Soc. Arts, Dec. 1979: 1–11.

54. ––––. 1981. The incidence of trace element deficiency diseases. Phil. Trans. R. Soc. Lond. B294:3–8.

55. U.S. Department of Agriculture. 1981. Agricultural statistics 1981. U.S. Government Printing Office, Washington, D.C.

56. Van Campen, D. R., and R. M. Welch. 1980. Availability to rats of iron from spinach: effects of oxalic acid. J. Nutr. 110:1618–1621.

57. Vohra, P., G. A. Gray, and F. H. Kratzer. 1965. Phytic acid-metal complexes. Proc. Soc. Exp. Biol. Med. 120:447–449.

58. Walker, C. D., and R. M. Welch. 1981. Low molecular weight metal compounds in edible plants. p. 155–157. In J. McC. Howell, J. M. Gawthorne, and C. L. White (ed.) Trace element metabolism in man and animals. Austral. Acad. Sci., Canberra.

59. Welch, R. M., and W. A. House. 1982. Availability to rats of zinc from soybean seeds as affected by maturity of seed, source of dietary protein, and soluble phytate. J. Nutr. 112:879–885.

60. ––––, ––––, and W. H. Allaway. 1974. Availability of zinc from pea seeds to rats. J. Nutr. 104:733–740.

61. ––––, ––––, and D. Van Campen. 1977. Effects of oxalic acid on availability of zinc from spinach leaves and zinc sulfate to rats. J. Nutr. 107:929–933.

62. ––––, and D. R. Van Campen. 1975. Iron availability to rats from soybeans. J. Nutr. 105:253–256.

63. West, T. S. 1981. Soil as the source of trace elements. Phil. Trans. R. Soc. Lond. B294: 19–39.

64. Widdowson, E. M. 1980. Man and the major mineral elements. p. 215–232. In K. Blaxter (ed.) Food chains and human nutrition. Applied Science Publishers Ltd., London.

65. Wright, M. J., and S. A. Ferrari (ed.) 1976. Plant adaptation to mineral stress in problem soils. Proceedings of a Workshop, Beltsville, Md., Nov. 22–23, 1976. Cornell Univ. Agric. Exp. Stn., Ithaca, N.Y.

66. Young, V. R., and M. Janghorbani. 1981. Soy proteins in human diets in relation to bioavailability of iron and zinc: a brief overview. Cereal Chem. 58:12–18.

67. Zhu, L. 1981. Keshan disease. p. 514–517. In J. McC. Howell, J. M. Gawthorne, and C. L. White (ed.) Trace element metabolism in man and animals. Austral. Acad. Sci., Canberra.

Chapter 4

The Effects of Processing and Refining on Nutritional Value of Crops[1]

ROBERT O. NESHEIM[2]

Crops are the major source of nutrients for people. Crops provide food products which may be consumed directly as with fruits, vegetables, nuts, cereal grains, and legumes, or indirectly from animal products produced by using crops and crop materials, such as forage, cereal grains, oil seed meals, and by-products, which are not directly consumed in human diets. Agronomists, through their contributions to the development and improvement of new and improved crops, increased yields, greater efficiency of production, and better utilization of production resources, have a very significant stake in the feeding of the world's population. It is important that agronomists have an interest in the nutritive contributions of crops to aid in improving the value of their research efforts to the nutrition of humankind.

This chapter is designed to provide the agronomist with some understanding of the effects of processing on nutritional value of crops. It will discuss in general why crops are processed, the effects processing may have on nutritive value, and the significance of this information to the agronomist in planning research and the application of new knowledge to crop production.

[1] Presented at symposium on "Crops as Sources of Nutrients for Humans". Annual meetings, Am. Soc. of Agron., 2 Dec. 1982, Anaheim, CA.

[2] Vice president, Science and Technology, Research and Quality Assurance, Cambridge Plan International, 1441 Schilling Place, Salinas, CA 93901-4592.

For more detailed and specific information on the effect of processing on specific nutrients, several excellent references are listed at the end of this chapter.

Processing of crops for food is not a new phenomenon of our modern industrial society. Processing of raw agricultural products for use as food dates from the time food was first changed from its natural state by cooking, grinding, stripping of inedible portions, and the like. In the early days of food gathering and preparation, processing occurred in the home by the individual or family unit. Today much of the processing is carried on in modern, highly efficient food processing plants.

REASONS FOR PROCESSING

Crops are processed for a variety of reasons. The removal of inedible fractions, producing physical and functional changes, improving palatability and nutritional quality, increasing convenience, destroying antinutritive factors and harmful bacteria, and preserving food for later consumption are the principal reasons for processing. Many of these factors are interrelated. The milling of wheat (*Triticum aestivum* L.) to remove the coarser fractions enables the baking of lighter breads, cakes, or other products which are convenient and palatable. Removing the hulls from oats (*Avena sativa* L.) and rolling the groat removes an inedible fraction and enables the production of a highly palatable food; additional processing permits greater convenience in preparation by cooking in the bowl with boiling water. Extracting the oil from soybeans [*Glycine max* (L.) Merr.] and heat treating the residue destroys antinutritive factors (trypsin inhibitors) and improves palatability through inhibiting the development of rancidity and improving the flavor of the meal. Further processing can result in more concentrated protein products, with specific functional characteristics which have application in formulating highly nutritious food products. The major purpose of food processing is preservation for later consumption. The development of thermal processing (canning) was a major step in food preservation, permitting seasonal foods to be available throughout the year. The development of freezing, dehydration, freeze drying, and irradiation as additional methods of preservation provide a series of options to use to preserve products with differing quality attributes for use by consumers on a nonseasonal basis.

EFFECTS OF PROCESSING ON NUTRITIONAL VALUE

Processing has an effect on the nutritional value of products. In most instances, particularly where thermal processes are used, some nutrient loss is inevitable. The degree of loss that occurs is dependent upon the susceptibility of the nutrient, the type of process employed, and how well it is controlled. Excessive heat over prolonged periods of time causes nutrient losses, particularly in the heat-labile nutrients, such as vitamin C, thiamin, and vitamin A. Commercial processing usually includes controls which will establish conditions necessary for safe preservation without excessive processing. Fortunately the conditions which provide optimum color and texture to canned products, or blanching of fruits and vegetables with hot water or steam for enzyme inactivation in pretreatment of frozen products, are consistent with minimizing nutrient losses.

The effect of processing on nutrient content of food produced from crops cannot be judged solely on the basis of nutrient losses occurring during manufacture. Nutrient losses occur in the entire chain of harvesting, processing, transporting, distribution, and home preparation. What is important is the nutrient content at the time of consumption. Nutrient content at harvesting is dependent upon the growing conditions, fertilizing practices, and the stage of maturity at which the crop is harvested. This will vary for different crops and for different nutrients. Losses occur also from the time of harvest until the product is processed. Enzyme systems are activated in the harvesting process which then must be controlled by such steps as blanching the raw product in hot water or steam before canning or freezing, or by chilling or controlling the atmosphere in the case of fresh vegetables and fruits. Canning, freezing, and dehydrating produce initial losses, but continuing losses are minimized when products are stored or shipped under appropriate conditions and properly displayed in retail stores. Home storage is also important, as is the method of home cooking. More variation in nutrient losses is likely to occur as a result of home preparation than from other parts of the processing chain due to lack of knowledge concerning proper food preparation as well as inadequate controls to avoid excessive cooking. There is remarkably little difference in total nutrient content in foods processed by various methods when the foods are finally prepared and served in the home.

Nutrient losses may be classified on the basis of their being intentional, inevitable, or avoidable. Intentional losses occur during milling of cereals, trimming of vegetables, extracting fractions, such as oils, starches, sugars, and protein concentrates or isolates. Inevitable losses of certain nutrients, particularly vitamin C and thiamin, occur during such processes as cooking, blanching, canning, and sterilizing. Avoidable losses occur primarily due to inadequate controls during heat processing, freezing, or excessive trimming of product.

There are considerable differences in the susceptibility of various nutrients to processing losses. Vitamin C and thiamin are the most susceptible of the vitamins and are often used as indicator nutrients in studying nutrient losses in the processing of foods. Minerals are quite stable. The macronutrients Ca, P, and Mg are not appreciably affected by processing. Trace minerals, such as Cu, Zn, and Se, are more susceptible to losses by leaching either in the blanching process or into the packing medium of canned fruits and vegetables. If the packing fluid is discarded, some of the nutrients are lost to the consumer.

In milling of wheat flour, significant losses of both vitamins and minerals occur in the removal of the bran and germ. The greater the extraction, that is, the more bran and germ removed, the lower will be the content of vitamins and minerals in the flour.

Processing protein products has both positive and negative effects. Heating the protein material, as in the toasting of soybeans following oil extraction, destroys antinutritive factors, such as the trypsin inhibitor, which interferes with the ability of the animal or man to digest the protein. Excessive heating in the presence of reducing sugars and moisture will result in a browning reaction, which reduces the availability of lysine and therefore may reduce the quality of the protein in the product. This same browning reaction imparts favorable flavor characteristics to many baked and cooked foods and therefore also has desirable aspects in improving food acceptance.

The preceding has been a general discussion of the influence of processing on various crops. More detailed information can be found in the excellent reviews and books listed at the end of this chapter.

MAXIMIZING THE NUTRITIONAL QUALITY OF CROPS

The concern of the agronomist, food scientist, and nutritionist should be to maximize the nutrient contribution of crops for the purpose of assuring nutritional adequacy of diets and making efficient use of food supplies. Several factors contribute to maximizing nutrient contributions from crops.

Breeding or selection of crop varieties for important nutrients can add to the nutritional quality of the food supply. Emphasis should be on improving the nutrient content of a crop when this crop is a significant source of that nutrient in the diet. There is little point in increasing the vitamin C content of mushrooms, for example, when mushrooms make up such a small part of our normal diets. A 50% increase in content of vitamin C would make an insignificant increase in daily intake in the diet. On the other hand, a 50% increase in the vitamin C content of potatoes (*Solanum tuberosum* L.) could be significant through the contribution to usual dietary intake of vitamin C. Therefore, the plant breeder needs to work closely with nutritionists and food scientists to make certain the research emphasis to improve nutrient content of a product is properly placed.

Knowledge of the influence of growing conditions and stage of harvest on nutrient content is important. This will enable the development of cultural practices to optimize nutrient production and yields. Cooperative efforts between agronomists, food scientists, and nutritionists will enable the identification of important production and harvesting practices to bring products to the market at a time that optimizes yield, nutrient content, and market acceptance.

Coordination of efforts between agronomists, agricultural engineers, food scientists, and nutritionists is necessary to minimize harvesting losses —losses of the food product itself and also the nutrient content. Desirable crop characteristics and harvesting and post-harvesting handling procedures can significantly reduce food and nutrient losses. Developing crops which may resist harvest damage would be valuable only if important nutrient content and market acceptance factors were retained.

Food processors must develop processing conditions which produce safe products while retaining key nutrient content and acceptance factors to the point of delivery of product to the consumer. Therefore, agronomists need to maintain communications with researchers in the entire chain of food processing and delivery to ascertain that the benefits of their research are reflected to the end product user. A high-yielding variety of rice (*Oryza sativa* L.), for example, which has good harvesting characteristics, high nutritive value, and keeps well in storage will be of little value if its cooking characteristics and flavor are such that the rice consumer does not find it acceptable.

SUMMARY

Significant opportunities exist for soil and plant scientists to work with food scientists and nutritionists to optimize the content of important nutrients in crops by advancing knowledge in breeding, selection, growing, harvesting, and processing. With the growing demand for food production as a result of expanding world population, it is necessary that optimizing nutrient contributions from production resources be achieved. I believe that significant progress will be made through integrating research efforts in food production and processing in the decades ahead.

The following is a partial listing of sources of specific information concerning the effect of various processes on the nutritive value of different crops:

Bender, A. E. 1978. Food processing and nutrition. Academic Press, London, England.

Harris, R. S. et al. 1975. Nutritional evaluation of food processing. AVI Publications Co., Westport, Conn.

Institute of Food Technology, Expert Panel on Food Safety and Nutrition. 1974. The effects of food processing on nutritional values. Food Technol. 28:77.

Rechcijl, M., Jr. (ed.) 1982. Handbook of nutritive value of processed food: Vol. 1. Food for human use. CRC Publications Company, Boca Raton, Fla.

Tannenbaum, S. R. 1979. Nutritional and safety aspects of food processing. Marcel Dekker, New York City, N.Y.

White, P. L. et al. (ed.) 1974. Nutrients in processed foods. American Medical Association.

Chapter 5

Soil Fertility and Plant Nutrition Effects on the Nutritional Quality of Crops[1]

V. V. RENDIG[2]

Except for that very small portion produced via synthetic culture media, or derived from chemical synthesis, food for humans comes directly or indirectly from crops grown in soil. Thus, to some extent, the composition of human diets reflects characteristics of the soil in which food crops are grown. For some mineral elements, such as K and Ca, entry into food chains is in the same form as they are absorbed from the soil. Others, such as N and S undergo various changes during their assimilation by plants, and thus these nutrients in foods are at least chemically different than the form in which they were absorbed. With the exception of B, all elements considered essential for plant growth are also considered essential for humans. Also included in listings of mineral elements required by humans are several others, such as I, Cr, and Se, not now considered plant-essential.

The degree to which the composition of foods as consumed will be influenced by the soil in which the crop is grown varies with the kind (species and variety) of crop, the nature of the food chain, the levels at which the elements occur in a form accessible for the growing crop, and the extent to which the harvested crop is altered prior to its consumption as food.

---

[1] Presented at symposium on "Crops as Sources of Nutrients for Human". Annual meetings, Am. Soc. of Agron., 2 Dec. 1982, Anaheim, CA.

[2] Professor, Dep. of Land, Air, and Water Resources, Univ. of California, Davis, CA 95616.

Well documented cases of a clear relationship of soil factors to our health are sparse. Most often cited as an example is the lack of I in certain soils, and perhaps more importantly in the water supply, in some areas of the world, where shortages of this element in the diet have been associated with the disorder cretinism, manifested by dwarfism, deformities, and thyroid enlargement (goiter). Prevention of this deficiency is achieved effectively by supplementing the diet, commonly by use of iodized table salt.

In certain areas of the world, including regions in the United States, Fe-deficiency anemia has been associated with low levels of soil Fe available to crops. It is most likely to occur in certain segments of the population, including women of child-bearing age, children, and those experiencing heavy blood loss through injury, illness, or some metabolic disorder. Generally, correction and prevention of the occurrence of deficiencies of Fe are best accomplished through dietary supplements.

Recent concerns have been expressed about the possibilities of intakes of excessive amounts of soil-borne elements capable of causing toxicity in humans. Thus, crops grown on soils in areas used for disposal of industrial wastes may contain Cd at levels at which there is a possibility of toxicity amongst some individuals in the population (Ryan, 1980). Wide differences of opinion exist as to the extent of this hazard and to the need for regulations to minimize or prevent risks to human health from improper waste disposal.

In view of the aspects of the subject of the Symposium covered by other speakers, this presentation will focus on research indicating quality differences associated with the mineral nutrition of cereal crops. Primary consideration will be given to effects of soil N supply, but with some comments also in regard to S nutrition. If the projections of Pimental et al. (1975) prove to be correct, there will have to be large increases in cereal production in the future because of increases in population, and cereal grains will account for a greater proportion of human protein needs. To provide this need, greater quantities of fertilizer N will be required, and as the marked increase in cost of these materials continues, the production of as many kilograms of protein as possible from each kilogram of fertilizer N used will become increasingly important. Consideration of the consequences of any change in fertilization practices on crop quality certainly should be included.

Direct evidence of improved human nutrition by changing the nature of the proteins in grain has been provided by the responses obtained when grain from corn (*Zea mays* L.) containing the *opaque-2* (*o-2*) gene and that from its normal counterpart are compared as protein sources (Beeson, 1966). No comparable comparisons have been made using grains grown on N-deficient soils to which N fertilizers have been applied. Evaluations of such responses in terms of nutritional implications have been made in consideration of recognized dietary needs or in comparison with foods considered as providing protein of high quality. Small animals, most commonly rats, have been used in some cases for quality assay. The validity of the assumptions made regarding the nutritional needs of different kinds of experimental animals and of humans is of course always open to question. Findings in recent studies by Burns et al. (1982), involving determination of protein-efficiency ratios (PER) of casein, soy isolate, and wheat (*Triticum aestivum* L.) gluten, indicate that responses of rats (*Rattus* sp.) tended to result in overestimates of the value of low quality proteins for dogs (*Canis familiaris*).

The adult, human protein requirement is uncertain. N.S. Scrimshaw of the Massachusetts Institute of Technology, speaking at a recent meeting of the Agricultural and Food Chemistry Division of the American Chemical Society, reported a proposal by the FAO/WHO/UNU Expert Consultation that this requirement be increased from 0.57 to 0.75 g/kg body weight. It was stated that this protein should be of "high quality", and that "It (protein requirement) will be higher for individuals recovering from infections". Also, that "elderly persons require a higher dietary density of protein and other essential nutrients than do young adults", and "Contrary to current opinion, dietary protein continues to be used for protein synthesis even when calories are deficient".

YIELD AND COMPOSITION RESPONSES TO N FERTILIZATION

The results shown in Fig. 1 for rice (*Oryza sativa* L.) are typical of the kind of response observed when N fertilizer is applied to a soil that contains an amount of N insufficient for crop needs. The concentration of protein in the grain continues to increase with the amount of N applied beyond the amount needed to obtain a maximum yield.

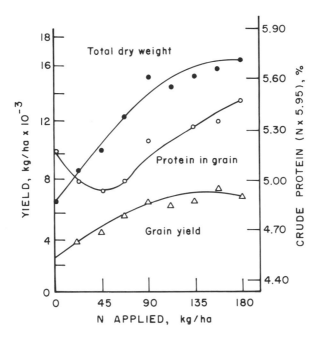

Fig. 1. Yields and protein concentrations of rice grown on a Stockton clay adobe soil with various rates of N applied (Miller and Mikkelsen, 1970).

Table 1. Levels of total N, nonprotein (NPN), and protein N in grain of wheat fertilized with
N at various levels (mean of six replicates, dry weight basis) (Dubetz et al., 1979).

Fertilizer N	Total N	NPN	Protein N†	NPN/total N
kg/ha		%		
0	2.19e‡	0.11d	2.08e	5.16c
50	2.41d	0.13cd	2.28d	5.34c
100	2.74c	0.14c	2.60c	5.22c
150	3.13b	0.17b	2.95b	5.46bc
200	3.27ab	0.19ab	3.08ab	5.87ab
250	3.34a	0.20a	3.14a	5.97ab
300	3.36a	0.21a	3.16a	6.17a
350	3.38a	0.20a	3.18a	5.94ab
400	3.37a	0.21a	3.16a	6.22a
Mean	3.02	0.17	2.85	5.70
SE	0.058	0.007	0.055	0.166

† Calculated by difference.
‡ a-e Values followed by the same letter within a column do not differ significantly (P
< 0.01).

A question raised by the indications shown in this response, as well as
other similar responses, is the validity of representing an increase in N
concentration as protein or crude protein. Upon treatment of most biological materials, including cereal grains, with the digestion mixture used
in the Kjeldahl-N analysis, at least a portion of the N present in constituents other than protein, including nitrate, are rendered to the am-
moniacal form and thus are included in the value calculated as protein.
Except for the possibility of some very unusual situations, for the analysis
of mature cereal grains the assumption that substantially all of the N is
present as protein generally does not lead to a large error in the estima-
tion. Even at a high rate of fertilization the relative proportion of nonprotein N is quite small (Table 1). Also, in most mature grains at least
some of the organic, nonprotein N would serve to some degree the same
purpose as protein in the nutrition of the consumer. Only a very small
fraction of the total would likely consist of nitrate-N. Use of other
methods specific for protein could eliminate this analytical problem.

EFFECTS OF N FERTILIZATION ON QUALITY
OF WHEAT GRAIN

Results of recent studies in North Dakota by Syltie et al. (1982) provide direct evidence of effects of N fertilization on crude protein concentrations and feeding quality of wheat (cv. Era and Waldron). The grain
for these studies was harvested from plots established at two different sites
in 2 successive years. At both sites the soils were mapped as the Heimdal
series (coarse-loamy, mixed Udic Haploborolls) but they differed in tex-
tural properties. Rats were fed ad lib for a period of 21 days using established procedures for such tests. As shown in Fig. 2, as the protein concentration in the grain increased the average daily gains of the animals increased and the feed required per unit of grain decreased. However, the

protein efficiency ratio (PER) calculated as the gain per unit of protein consumed, decreased with increases in protein concentration in the grain (Fig. 3). The protein digestibility coefficient (PDC), a measure of the fraction of the protein digested by the rats, increased significantly as protein concentrations increased for the wheats grown on the Heimdal loam but was not affected over the higher range of protein concentrations of the wheat grown at the other site. It was suggested that the higher PDC values could be the result of larger kernel size, resulting in higher proportions of the more digestible endosperm and embryo.

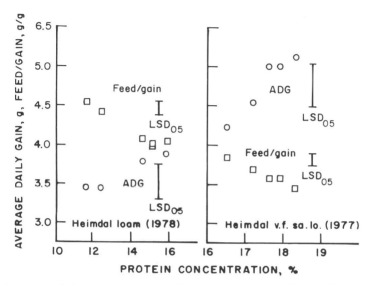

Fig. 2. Average daily gains and amounts of grain consumed per unit gain of rats fed grain containing different concentrations of protein (Syltie et al., 1982).

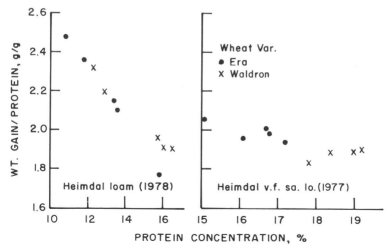

Fig. 3. Weight gains per unit protein consumed for rats fed grain differing in protein concentration (Syltie et al., 1982).

Table 2. Effects of N fertilization on total protein concentration and amounts of N in protein fractions of wheat grain (Dubetz et al., 1979).

Nitrogen	Protein conc.	Protein fractions				
		Albumin	Globulin	Gliadin	Glutenin 1	Glutenin 2
kg/ha	%	mg/100 g, dry wt. basis				
0	13.0e†	30.0	42.2	60.6	2.7	58.8
50	14.3d	33.3	42.1	86.8	4.0	72.7
100	16.3c	33.3	46.0	122.9	6.7	75.1
400	19.8a	34.4	51.7	143.3	6.4	75.6

† a-e Values within a column not having a common letter differ significantly (P < 0.01), based on calculations from data including N treatments of 150, 200, 250, 300, and 350 kg/ha.

The decreases in PER values associated with the increases in protein concentration for the wheat grown at the Heimdal loam site were attributed by Syltie et al. to lower concentrations of a growth-limiting amino acid in the protein, most likely lysine. This was documented by citations from earlier investigations with barley (*Hordeum vulgare* L.) (Sure, 1954). This view is also supported by the more recent findings of Dubetz and Gardiner (1979). They grew wheat (cv. Neepawa) in Alberta (Can.) on plots to which N as ammonium nitrate was applied at rates ranging from 0 to 300 kg/ha and urea spray at 0 to 100 kg/ha with six replications of each treatment. Highly significant decreases in the concentration in the protein of lysine as well as histidine, aspartic acid, and threonine, and increases in concentrations of glutamic acid and proline, were found with increasing rates of applications of both fertilizers. Increases in phenylalanine were found with both kinds of applied N but this was highly significant only with the urea spray. It is noted that three of the four amino acids which showed decreases in concentration are considered, by the pathway of their biosynthesis in plants, to be members of the aspartate family (Bryan, 1976).

In earlier studies with the Neepawa wheat, Dubetz et al. (1979) had also found highly significant increases associated with increasing rates of N application for glutamate, proline, and phenylalanine. However, unlike the results from the later studies, threonine again, as well as serine, glycine, and alanine showed decreases in concentration. Data obtained from fractionation of the protein by solubility differences indicated that the main effect of N application was a decrease in the gliadin fraction (Table 2). From this response and the data provided for the amino acid analysis of the various protein fractions (Table 3), predictions as to changes in amino acid concentrations that would likely occur with additions of N can be made. Thus, glutamate, proline, and phenylalanine would be expected to increase, and lysine, arginine, aspartate, threonine, serine, glycine, and alanine to decrease. Dubetz et al. stated in their paper that, while the concentration of lysine in the wheat from the plots to which 400 kg/ha was added was 18% less than with no added N, this was not statistically significant. Also in these studies compared to those done subsequently, a larger number (9) of application rates were used, but the concentration of N in the grain changed very little beyond the third 50-kg increment.

Table 3. The amino acid composition of protein fractions in wheat grain
(means of four N treatments) (Dubetz et al., 1979).

| | Protein fractions | | | | | |
Amino acid	Albumin	Globulin	Gliadin	Glutenin 1	Glutenin 2	SE
			Mole % on an ammonia-free basis			
Lysine	4.8a†	5.1a	0.7c	1.2c	2.1b	0.10
Histidine	2.2b	3.1a	1.8b	0.9c	0.6c	0.15
Arginine	5.2b	10.7a	2.0d	3.5c	4.3bc	0.25
Aspartate	7.7a	8.0a	2.6d	4.0c	5.4b	0.16
Threonine	3.8a	3.8a	1.7d	2.5c	3.0b	0.11
Serine	4.0ab	4.5a	2.9c	4.4a	3.4bc	0.16
Glutamate	24.6c	19.2d	42.3a	41.7a	35.0b	0.77
Proline	9.4c	4.8d	15.0a	12.0b	9.9c	0.39
Glycine	4.2b	5.4a	1.6c	3.8b	4.9a	0.13
Alanine	5.1a	5.2a	1.8d	2.4c	3.6b	0.07
Cystine (half)	2.8a	2.2ab	2.4a	1.3bc	1.0c	0.22
Valine	6.1a	6.5a	4.2bc	3.5c	4.7b	0.22
Methionine	1.9a	2.0a	1.3b	1.3b	1.8a	0.12
Isoleucine	3.3b	3.9a	3.8	3.4b	3.7a	0.06
Leucine	7.2b	7.4b	6.6c	6.6c	7.9a	0.11
Tyrosine	2.6c	3.2b	2.8bc	3.2b	4.4a	0.10
Phenylalanine	4.9bc	4.6c	6.0a	5.4b	4.8c	0.12

† a-d Values within a row, not having common letter differ significantly (P < 0.01).

EFFECT OF N FERTILIZATION ON QUALITY OF CORN GRAIN

Effects on weight gains of rats have been obtained with corn grain from plots grown in plots with various levels of N applied (Table 4). (Ishibashi, D. 1978. The effects of N fertilization on the nutritional quality of corn grain. M.S. Thesis, Univ. of California, Davis.) Groups of five individually housed rats were fed one of seven diets for a period of 21 days. It does not appear that the low weight gains of the rats fed corn grain was limited by the level of protein in the ration since better gains were obtained at the same protein levels from the lactalbumin and starch ration (Table 4a). There seems to be no apparent explanation for the much higher level of urinary N excretion from the rats fed the grain from the plots fertilized at the 180 N level. The N fertilization level under which the crop was grown had a greater effect on the accumulation of body fat energy than on the retention of protein (Table 4b). Calculation of adjusted energy deposition coefficients (Canolty and Koong, 1976) indicated differences in retention for the grain grown at the several N fertilization levels (Table 4c).

Based on total protein present, the concentrations of four amino acids generally recognized as being nutritionally essential or beneficial (i.e., tryptophan, lysine, threonine, and arginine) decreased significantly as the level of N applied to the corn crop increased, and one essential amino acid, phenylalanine, increased (Table 5). Of those amino acids not considered essential, glycine showed a decrease in concentration in the protein with increases in rates of N fertilization, while four, alanine, tyrosine, glutamate (includes glutamine), and leucine increased in concentrations.

Based on the weight of grain, the concentrations of all amino acids increased as the amount of fertilizer N applied was increased. However, the concentrations of tryptophan, lysine, glycine, arginine, and threonine showed less increase than did the concentration of crude protein, while others, notably, glutamate (includes glutamine), proline and leucine, increased more than did crude protein. Thus, when calculated on the basis of protein, three amino acids considered nutritionally essential, tryptophan, lysine, and threonine, decreased significantly and one, phenylalanine, increased significantly with treatment.

Table 4. Effects of N fertilization of corn on quality of grain by rate growth assay method (121 day), (Ishibashi, D. 1978. The effects of N fertilization on the nutritional quality of corn grain. M.S. Thesis, Univ. of Calif., Davis).

(a) Weight gains and protein utilization

Ration[†]	Crude protein	Wt. Wt. gains	Net protein utilization	Urinary[§] N excretion
		%		mg
Corn (0N)	4.68	3.5 ± 2.5	46.2 ± 4.1	42.3 ± 7.6
Corn (90N)	5.29	6.1 ± 1.1	42.6 ± 4.4	58.6 ± 15.6
Corn (180N)	6.81	4.6 ± 0.5	44.5 ± 1.9	118 ± 6.3
Corn (360N)	7.41	10.4 ± 2.9	52.5 ± 2.1	80.5 ± 15.4
Syn A[‡]	3.26	4.0 ± 1.5	69.4 ± 1.9	20.8 ± 1.7
Syn B	4.76	14.8 ± 3.9	77.1 ± 2.0	19.0 ± 3.5
Syn C	7.32	24.3 ± 1.9	77.2 ± 2.2	4.5 ± 7.8

(b) Changes in body protein and carcass fat levels.

Ration[†] (rate of N fert.)	Change in body protein	Change in carcass fat energy
Corn (0N)	3.14 ± 0.39	22.7 ± 6.8
Corn (90N)	4.54 ± 0.44	24.3 ± 5.4
Corn (180N)	4.82 ± 0.49	3.04 ± 7.8
Corn (360N)	5.04 ± 0.37	10.1 ± 7.2
Syn A[‡]	2.54 ± 0.26	62.7 ± 8.8
Syn B	4.67 ± 0.50	45.6 ± 17.2
Syn C	8.34 ± 0.53	6.4 ± 1.4

(c) Deposition of energy relative to grain protein.

Ration[†]	Adjusted energy deposition coefficients[¶]	
	Lean	Fat
Corn (0N)	2.4 ± 0.5	6.9 ± 0.8
Corn (90N)	2.8 ± 0.3	6.9 ± 0.9
Corn (180N)	1.5 ± 0.2	3.2 ± 0.6
Corn (360N)	1.7 ± 0.2	3.4 ± 0.6
Syn A[‡]	2.9 ± 0.5	12.0 ± 1.2
Syn B	1.8 ± 0.4	6.5 ± 1.2
Syn C	1.7 ± 0.4	2.3 ± 0.5

† In addition to salt mix and vitamins. Figures in parentheses are levels (kg/ha) of N applied to plots on which corn was grown.
‡ Lactalbumin and starch.
§ During 3-day test period.
¶ Kcal deposited in lean and fat per kcal of available dietary protein (Canolty and Koong, 1976).

Fractionation of the protein in the corn grain by a modified Osborne-Mendel procedure (Paulis et al., 1975) revealed that the main effect of N fertilization was the increase in concentration of the prolamine (zein) fraction (Table 6). Similar observations had been made in earlier studies (Keeney, 1970; Kohnke and Vestal, 1948; MacGregor et al., 1961; Sauberlich et al., 1953). Ever since early in this century it has been known that for experimental animals being fed a ration with zein as a protein source, additions of lysine and tryptophan were necessary for the animals to grow well. Results typical of those obtained in a number of these early experiments are shown in Fig. 4 (Osborne and Mendel, 1914).

Whether all of the plant N supply-related difference in nutritional quality of grains, as indicated by responses such as described above with rat growth assays, can be attributed to effects on protein distribution is not certain. While some of the differences in composition of the corn

Table 5. Effects of N fertilization on the concentrations of amino acids in the protein and of protein N in maize (Pioneer 3780) grain (Rendig and Broadbent, 1979).

Amino acids	Concentrations of amino acids in grain from plants grown with four rates (kg ha^{-1}) of N application				
	0	90	180	360	
	— mg amino acid N/(100 mg protein N) —				
Tryptophan	3.61a	2.74a	1.49b	1.47b	
Lysine	4.94a	4.34a	3.73b	3.57b	
Glycine	7.11a	6.47b	5.67c	5.73c	
Arginine	12.99a	11.80b	11.06c	11.18c	
Aspartic acid	6.20	5.84	5.88	5.83	NS†
Threonine	3.61a	3.38b	3.37b	3.34b	
Serine	5.37	5.36	5.42	5.50	NS
Valine	3.88	4.03	3.75	3.98	NS
Histidine	5.62	5.65	5.44	5.48	NS
Methionine	1.48	1.67	1.60	1.42	NS
Isoleucine	2.27	2.45	2.33	2.61	NS
Proline	8.13	8.62	9.08	8.48	NS
Alanine	8.54a	8.68a	9.24b	9.27b	
Tyrosine	2.15a	2.40b	2.48b	2.36b	
Phenylalanine	2.46a	2.83b	2.90bc	3.00c	
Glutamic acid	12.31a	13.03b	14.52c	14.27c	
Leucine	7.83a	8.79b	10.03c	10.21c	

† a-c values within a row not having a common letter differ significantly (P < 0.05).

Table 6. Effects of amounts of N fertilization of corn on the concentrations of protein fractions extracted from the grain (from Rendig and Broadbent, 1979).

N applied	Albumin-globulin	Zein	Alcohol soluble glutelin	Residue†
kg/ha	— % of dry wt. as N —			
0	0.27a‡	0.14a	0.29a	0.26a
90	0.32a	0.24b	0.30a	0.16a
180	0.30a	0.48c	0.36b	0.46b
360	0.33a	0.58d	0.35b	0.39b

† Includes alcohol-insoluble glutelin.
‡ a-d values in a column not having a common letter differ significantly (P < 0.05).

Table 7. Ratios of concentrations of amino acids (as mg amino acid N/100 mg protein N) in zein to those in whole grain (zein data from sources indicated, whole grain data from Rendig and Broadbent, 1979).

Amino acid	Mosse (1966)	Jimenez (1966)
Leucine	1.76	1.78
Phenylalamine	1.59	1.59
Glutamic acid	1.34	1.43
Alanine	1.37	1.43
Isoleucine	1.33	1.57
Serine	1.13	1.13
Proline	1.07	1.11
Valine	1.03	1.01
Threonine	0.83	0.87
Aspartic acid	0.79	0.89
Methionine	0.73	0.66
Histidine	0.51	0.53
Arginine	0.45	0.35
Glycine	0.40	0.39
Lysine	0.03	0.06

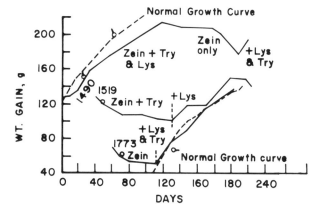

Fig. 4. Growth of rats fed zein alone or supplemented with lysine and/or tryptophan (Osborne and Mendel, 1914).

grain, grown at different levels of N supply, are consistent with the observed higher proportion of zein, others are not. As a test of whether or not the effects on the zein fraction account for the response to N fertilization of increased protein concentration overall, the concentrations of amino acids in zein and in the whole grain were compared. Using data obtained from field plot studies for the grain analyses (Rendig and Broadbent, 1979) and published zein data (Mosse, 1966; Jimenez, 1966), ratios of the two values were calculated (Table 7). Increases from N fertilization that this comparison would predict are for leucine, glutamic acid, pheylalanine, alanine, isoleucine, serine, and proline. As described previously, this was noted for the first four but not for the other three. Likewise, decreases would be predicted for tryptophan, lysine, glycine, argin-

Table 8. Effects of N fertilization on the contents of lysine and tryptophan, and the chemical score of grain proteins. Amino acids as grain amino acid per 16 g N (Breteler, 1976).

Nitrogen applied	Lysine		Tryptophan		Chemical score†	
	CIV-2	0-2	CIV-2	0-2	CIV-2	0-2
kg/ha	——— g amino acids/16 g N ———					
35	3.8	5.1	0.83	0.91	53	61
60	2.1	3.9	0.80	0.90	29	54
104	2.0	3.5	0.84	0.86	28	49
207	2.0	3.6	0.70	0.87	38	50
276	1.9	2.7	0.68	0.88	26	38
2 x 38	1.6	1.9	0.58	0.82	22	26

† With reference to whole egg protein.

ine, threonine, aspartate, valine, and histidine. This was not noted for the latter three, but was for the others.

The studies of Hogan et al. (1955) also showed that rats grew poorly on corn unless it was supplemented by lysine and tryptophan. In these studies, growth responses with corn from two sources, and containing 16.1 and 7.3% protein, were compared. Better weight gains were obtained with the higher protein corn, whether or not amino acid supplements were added alone or in combination to the rations. However, a higher biological value of the protein in the low-protein corn was indicated by greater gains and better feed efficiency per unit of protein eaten. A higher "calorie gain/protein intake" was indicated for the low-protein corn but the method by which this calculation was made was not described. The best mean weight gain (94.9 g) obtained with the corn-based rations were somewhat less than that (117.4 g) obtained with a casein ration.

There is no clear evidence whether the increased levels of grain protein leucine associated with the application of higher rates of N have any significant effect on grain quality. While leucine is an essential amino acid, it also has been implicated as a factor in increasing urinary excretion of N-methyl-nicotinamide (Gopolan et al., 1969), and as a competitive inhibitor in the intestinal absorption of tryptophan (Sakakihara. 1982).

Results obtained in feeding studies with rats (Mertz et al., 1964) and with humans (Beeson, 1966) have shown that the quality of corn grain can be improved by incorporation of the recessive mutant gene, o-2. Similarly as for the normal counterparts, the grain protein of the genetically modified genotype reflects the level of N with which the crop is grown. With the genotypes used by Breteler (1976), decreases in lysine were much greater than for tryptophan (Table 8). Chemical scores calculated with reference to egg protein indicated that at the lowest N level used, tryptophan would be the limiting amino acid, but with higher rates of application of N, lysine would be limiting. These responses could be different for other genotypes. Biological values calculated with reference to human milk have shown lysine and tryptophan to be about equally limiting in corn grain (Wokes, 1968; Young, 1976). As with any other dietary con-

Table 9. Effects of various levels of applied N on the yields of crude protein and amino acids (Rendig and Broadbent, 1979).

Applied N	Crude protein	Tryptophan	Lysine	Leucine
		kg/ha		
0	421a†	13a	13a	38a
90	512b	17a	19b	67b
180	1028c	18a	32c	154c
360	1016c	17a	30c	155c

† a-c values in a column not having a common letter differ significantly (P < 0.05).

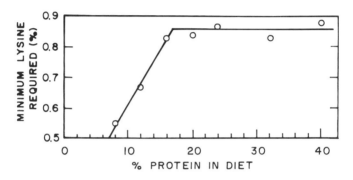

Fig. 5. Lysine requirement for rats as related to the concentration of protein in the diet (Rosenberg, 1957).

stituent, the level of an amino acid required for nutritional needs is influenced by various factors. The data in Fig. 5 show the increased level of dietary lysine required for growth of rats on an isocaloric ration as the level of protein increases.

The amounts of protein and amino acids produced per unit land area are important considerations in evaluating influences of N fertilization on plant composition in terms of nutritional quality. The data obtained from the corn studies previously described are shown in Table 9. Because the different forms of protein in the grain are affected differently as described above, the effects of N treatments on the yields of individual amino acids will not be the same as for total protein. Thus, as the rate of N applied was increased, tryptophan increased much less than lysine or leucine, when calculated on the basis of land area.

COMPARATIVE RESPONSES FOR CEREAL GRAINS

Effects of N fertilization on grain protein quality can also be expressed in terms of the ratio of essential to nonessential amino acids (Table 10). Although the values obtained from data reported in the literature

Table 10. Effects of N nutrition on the ratios of essential to nonessential amino acids in some varieties of cereal grains.

Crop	Fertilizer treatments Lo N†		Hi N‡	Grain yield Increases	Protein concentrations§ Lo N	Hi N	Amino acid ratios: Essential/nonessential Lo N	Hi N	References¶
					%				
Barley									
Lofa	1	g/pot	12	94	9.09	17.5	0.88	0.73	4
Impala	1.5 g/pot		5	114	9.21	14.8	0.88	0.76	3
Wheat									
Kleiber	1	g/pot	12	36	9.00	16.7	0.78	0.67	4
Neepawa	0	kg/ha	300	3	17.7	20.7	0.53	0.51	1
Neepawa	0	kg/ha	400	145	13.7	20.7	0.63	0.62	2
Spring rye (*Secale cereale*)									
Petkus	1	g/pot	4	(67)#	7.75	10.6	0.91	0.80	5
Petkus	1	g/pot	12	(1)	7.75	17.6	0.91	0.71	5
Oats									
Selma	1	g/pot	10	(136)	5.95	13.1	1.01	1.01	5
Rice (milled)									
Saturn/									
Bluebell	0	kg/ha	134	55	6.23	6.65	1.15	0.99	7
Corn									
PX-20	2.4 g/pot		9.6	203	5.20	9.67	0.97	0.94	8
Pioneer 3780	0	kg/ha	360	82	5.56	9.60	0.88	0.86	9
Wis. 1710	0	kg/ha	200	1060	6.5	8.3	0.91	0.90	6
Wis. 1718	0	kg/ha	200	400	5.8	6.8	0.93	0.88	6
Wis. 273	0	kg/ha	200	360	7.9	7.6	0.91	0.94	6

† Lo N = N applied at lowest rate used.
‡ Hi N = N applied at highest rate used.
§ Calculated from conversion factors given in Watt and Merrill (1963).
¶ References: (1) Dubetz and Gardiner, 1979; (2) Dubetz et al., 1979; (3) Eppendorfer, 1968; (4) Eppendorfer, 1975; (5) Eppendorfer, 1977; (6) Keeney, 1970; (7) Patrick and Hoskins, 1974; (8) Perez-Zamora, 1979. Effects of nitrogen and phosphorus additions on the growth and composition of corn plants grown on a calcareous soil. Ph.D. Thesis, Univ. of California; (9) Rendig and Broadbent, 1979.
# ( ) Total dry matter; grain yields not given.

show some exceptions, wheat, barley, and rye (*Secale cereale* L.) show the greatest effect. For oats (*Avena sativa* L.) and the Neepawa wheat, there were no differences between grain grown with two different levels of N applied. The lack of an effect in the case of corn grain seems most likely explained by noting (Table 5) that leucine, an essential amino acid, is increased sufficiently by addition of N so that the ratio of essential amino acids to nonessential does not change. In making these kind of comparisons with data from different sources, caution should be exercised against over generalization.Differences in sampling, handling of samples and methods of analysis can obscure and exaggerate differences. As pointed out by Patrick et al. (1974), the rice data shown in Table 10 are for grain which has been milled, and in the process would lose a portion of the kernel that would likely have a higher lysine concentration than would the remaining endosperm.

Table 1. Effects of different concentrations of total-N, cystine, and methionine of seed
Vicia faba on true digestibility (TD), biological value (BV) and net protein
utilization (NPU) (Eppendorfer, 1971).

S/pot	Total-N	Cystine	Methionine	TD	BV	NPU
g	%	—g amino acid/16 g N—			Mean ± S.D.†	
0	3.97	0.95	0.80	80.8 ± 2.3	40.8 ± 2.1	33.0 ± 2.6
0.25	4.24	1.26	0.87	84.3 ± 2.6	55.5 ± 2.6	47.1 ± 2.7
1.00	4.32	1.38	0.87	84.7 ± 1.4	60.2 ± 2.4	51.0 ± 2.4
4.00	4.25	1.53	0.89	85.0 ± 1.7	58.0 ± 2.2	49.3 ± 2.3
0‡	3.97	1.52	0.89	80.7 ± 2.2	53.5 ± 2.1	43.2 ± 2.1

† SD = Standard deviation.
‡ Cystine and methionine contents of dry matter at the 0 S level was increased to those of the
4.0 g S level by addition of synthetic cystine and methionine.

EFFECTS OF S FERTILIZATION ON SEED QUALITY

Since S is a structural element of three amino acids, methionine, cysteine, and cystine, it might be expected that the composition of at least some part of plants grown in soils containing insufficient amounts of S could be affected if additional fertilizer S was applied. Increases in the concentration of cyst(e)ine (reported as cystine but also included cysteine) in protein by a maximum of about 50%, with smaller increases in methionine, were found in greenhouse studies with field beans (*Vicia faba*) grown on soil to which different levels of S was applied (Eppendorfer, 1971). Results from feeding experiments with rats showed significant increases in true digestibility (TD), biological value (BV) and net protein utilization (NPU) (Table 11). Additions of cystine and methionine to the low-S seeds from the high-S treatment had no effect on TD but did increase the BV and NPU, not to the values found for the rats fed the high-S seeds, however.

Results from a limited number of studies involving the relationship of nutrient S levels to specific proteins and protein fractions have shown some effects similar to those with N. Moss et al. (1981) found that lower concentrations of S in wheat flour were associated with lower proportions of albumin and higher proportions of those gliadins showing low mobility in electrophoretic separation and containing lesser amounts of cysteine and methionine (Fig. 6). These differences were most marked in samples from plants grown with an abundant N supply and with flour S concentrations below about 0.11%.

Similar results have been reported for other species. Blagrove et al. (1976) found that the proportions of different forms of the globulin protein fraction in lupin (*Lupinus augustifolius* L.) seeds were affected by the level of S under which the plants were grown. Under such conditions, seeds of blue lupin and in subsequent studies (Gillespie et al., 1978) seeds of other species of lupin as well, contained higher concentrations of conglutin β, and lower concentrations of the α and γ forms. The β form contains no methionine and very low amounts of cyst(e)ine. Additional research is needed to determine whether this kind of response, which could be very important from the standpoint of crop quality, is a general

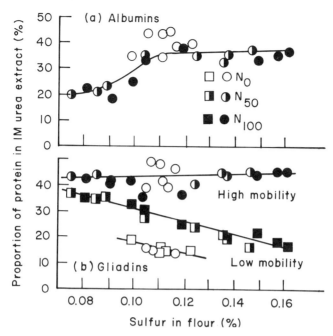

Fig. 6. Proportions of protein in wheat grain present as albumin and gliadins as related to S concentration in the flour (Moss et al., 1981).

one in other plants of which seeds are used as food. Cyst(e)ine, though not one of the amino acids considered as essential, is important in quality considerations because of its sparing action for methionine. In studies using five varieties of dry beans (*Phaseolus vulgaris* L.), and one variety of mung bean [*Vigna unguiculata* (L.) Walp.] differing in S contents, Porter et al. (1974) found that PER correlated significantly with the sum of cystine and methionine but not with either amino acid alone.

SUMMARY AND CONCLUSIONS

The evidence reviewed here indicates that the makeup of proteins in cereal grains as well as other seeds is influenced by N and S nutrition of the growing crop, and that these changes can influence the utilization of proteins by the consumer. Whether or not these responses merit consideration in developing fertilizer management practices is uncertain. It has been demonstrated that changes in protein distribution and amino acid balance can be achieved through plant breeding, and this may well be the better approach. However, as pointed out by Hanson (1979) and as still prevails, there is as yet insufficient information about the N harvest index and its relationship to N acquisition and remobilization to apply this knowledge to crop breeding. A better understanding of crop physiology is necessary also in seeking genotypes possessing the desirable stability of grain protein amino acid composition under different nutritional regimes.

ACKNOWLEDGMENT

The author acknowledges with thanks permission from the Agricultural Institute of Canada to use the data of Tables 2, 3, and 4 from the *Canadian Journal of Plant Science*, and the CSIRO Editorial and Publication Service to use Fig. 6 from the *Australian Journal of Agricultural Research*.

REFERENCES

1. Beeson, W. M. 1966. Feed and Food value of *opaque-2*. Proc. 21st Corn Research Conf., American Seed Trade Association.

2. Blagrove, R. J., J. M. Gillespie, and P. J. Randall. 1976. Effect of sulphur supply on seed globulin composition of *Lupinus angustifolium*. Aust. J. Plant Physiol. 3:173–184.

3. Breteler, H. 1976. Nitrogen fertilization, yield and protein quality of a normal and high-lysine maize variety. J. Sci. Food Agric. 27:978–982.

4. Bryan, J. K. 1976. Amino acid biosynthesis and its regulation. *In* J. Bonner and J. E. Varner (ed.) Plant biochemistry. 3rd ed. Academic Press, Inc., New York.

5. Burns, R. A., M. H. LeFaivre, and J. A. Milner. 1982. Effects of dietary protein quantity and quality on the growth of dogs and rats. J. Nutr. 112:1843–1853.

6. Canolty, N. L., and L. J. Koong. 1976. Utilization of energy for maintenance and for fat and lean gains by mice selected for rapid postweaning growth rates. J. Nutr. 106:1202–1208.

7. Dubetz, S., and E. E. Gardiner. 1979. Effect of nitrogen fertilizer treatments on amino acid composition of Neepawa wheat. Cereal Chem. 56:166–168.

8. ————, ————, D. Flynn, and A. Ian De La Roche. 1979. Effect of nitrogen fertilizer on nitrogen fractions and amino acid composition of spring wheat. Can. J. Plant Sci. 59: 299–305.

9. Eppendorfer, W. 1968. The effect of nitrogen and sulphur on changes in nitrogen fractions of barley plants at various stages of growth and on yield and amino acid composition of grain. Plant Soil 29:424–438.

10. ————. 1971. Effects of S, N, and P on amino acid composition of field beans (*Vicia faba*) and responses of the biological value of the seed protein to S-amino acid content. J. Sci. Food Agric. 22:501–505.

11. ————. 1975. Effects of fertilizers on quality and nutritional value of grain protein. *In* Int. Potash Inst. Fertilizer Use and Protein Production, 11th Colloquium, Berne, Switzerland.

12. ————. 1977. Nutritive value of oat and rye grain protein as influenced by nitrogen and amino acid composition. J. Sci. Food Agric. 28:152–156.

13. Gillespie, J. M., R. J. Blagrove, and P. J. Randall. 1978. Effect of sulfur supply on the seed globulin composition of various species of lupin. Aust. J. Plant Physiol. 5:641–650.

14. Gopolan, C., B. Belevady, and D. Krishnamurthi. 1969. The role of leucine in the pathogenesis of canine black-tongue and pellagra. Lancet 11:956–957.

15. Hanson, A. 1979. Plant breeding and partitioning in cereals and grain legumes. *In* Michigan State Univ. Partitioning of assimilates. Summary reports of a workshop.

16. Hogan, A. G., G. T. Gillespie, O. Kocturk, G. L. O'Dell, and L. M. Flynn. 1955. The percentage of protein in corn and its nutritional properties. J. Nutr. 57:225–239.

17. Jimenez, J. R. 1966. Protein fractionation studies of high lysine corn. Proc. High Lysine Corn Conference, Purdue Univ., Lafayette, Ind.

18. Keeney, D. R. 1970. Protein and amino acid composition of maize grain as influenced by variety and fertility. J. Sci. Food Agric. 12:182–184.

19. Kohnke, H., and C. M. Vestal. 1948. The effect of nitrogen fertilization on the feeding value of corn. Soil Sci. Soc. Am. Proc. 13:299–302.

20. MacGregor, J., L. T. Taskovitch, and W. P. Martin. 1961. Effect of nitrogen fertilizer and soil type on the amino acid content of corn grain. Agron. J. 53:211–216.

21. Mertz, E. T., L. S. Bates, and O. E. Nelson. 1964. Mutant gene that changes protein composition and increases lysine content of maize endosperm. Science 145:279–280.

22. Miller, M. D., and D. S. Mikkelsen. 1970. 1969 rice and seed protein studies. Rice J. 73: 38–42.

23. Moss, H. J., C. W. Wrigley, F. MacRitchie, and P. J. Randall. 1981. Sulfur and nitrogen fertilizer effects on wheat. II. Influence on grain quality. Aust. J. Agric. Res. 32: 213–226.

24. Mosse, J. 1966. Alcohol-soluble proteins of cereal grains. Fed. Proc. 25:1666–1669.

25. Osborne, T. B., and L. B. Mendel. 1914. Amino-acids in nutrition and growth. J. Biol. Chem. XVII:325–355.

26. Patrick, R. M., F. H. Hoskins, E. Wilson, and F. J. Peterson. 1974. Protein and amino acid content of rice as affected by application of nitrogen fertilizer. Cereal Chem. 51: 84–95.

27. Paulis, J.W., J. A. Bietz, and J. S. Wall. 1975. Corn protein subunits: molecular weights determined by sodium dodecyl sulfate-polyacrylamide gel electrophoresis. Agric. Food Chem. 23:197–201.

28. Perez-Zamora, O. 1979. Effects of nitrogen and phosphorus addition on the growth and composition of corn (Zea mays L.) grown on a calcareous soil. Ph.D. Thesis, Univ. of Calif., Davis, Calif.

29. Pimentel, D., W. Dritschilo, J. Krummel, and J. Kutzman. 1975. Energy and land constraints in food protein production. Science 190:754–761.

30. Porter, W. M., J. H. Maner, J. D. Axtell, and W. F. Keim. 1974. Evaluation of the nutritive quality of grain legumes by an analysis for total sulfur. Crop Sci. 11:652–654.

31. Randall, P. J., K. Spencer, and J. R. Freney. 1981. Sulfur and nitrogen fertilizer effects on wheat. I. Concentrations of sulfur and nitrogen and the nitrogen to sulfur ratio in grain, in relation to the yield response. Aust. J. Agric. Res. 32:203–212.

32. Rendig, V. V., and F. E. Broadbent. 1979. Proteins and amino acids in grain of maize grown with various levels of applied N. Agron. J. 71:509–512.

33. Rosenberg, H. R. 1957. Methionine and lysine supplementation of animal feeds. J. Agric. Food Chem. 5:696–700.

34. Ryan, J. A. 1980. Analysis of the cadmium issue. Resource Use Committee of the Fertilizer Institute.

35. Sakakibara, S., K. Jugii, S. Nasu, H. Imai, K. Yamaguchi, and I. Ueda. 1982. Effect of L-leucine-supplemented diet on the nicotine amide adenine dinucleotide content of rat liver. J. Nutr. 112:1688–1695.

36. Sauberlich, H. E., Wan-Yuin Chang, and W. D. Salmon. 1953. The amino acid and protein content of corn as related to variety and nitrogen fertilization. J. Nutr. 51:241–250.

37. Sure, B. 1954. Influence of lysine, valine, and threonine additions on the efficiency of protein of whole wheat. Arch. Biochem. Biophys. 39:463–464.

38. Syltie, P. W., W. C. Dahnke, and R. L. Harrold. 1982. Nutritional value of hard red spring wheat grain protein as influenced by fertilization and cultivar. Agron. J. 74:366–371.

39. Watt, B. K., and A. L. Merrill. 1963. Composition of foods. Agric. Handb. No. 8, USDA.

40. Wokes, F. 1968. Proteins. Plant Foods Hum. Nutr. 1:23–42.

41. Young, R. E. 1976. Protein requirements-quantity and quality. In B. H. Beard and M. H. Miller (ed.) Opportunities to improve protein quality and quantity for human food. Univ. of California Div. Agric. Sci. Spec. Pub. 3058.

Chapter 6

Potential for Improved Crop Nutritional Quality in Cereals through Plant Breeding[1]

V. A. JOHNSON[2]

Plants, directly or indirectly, provide essentially all of the world's food. As world population continues to increase, direct consumption of plants as food also must increase because most plants are more efficient producers of calories and protein than are animals. An exception is the conversion of forages by ruminant animals into food that can be digested by man.

Cereals are the most important food plant group. It has been estimated that wheat (*Triticum aestivum* L.) and rice (*Oryza sativa* L.) alone are dietary mainstays for approximately two-thirds of all people on earth. Maize (*Zea mays* L.), sorghum [*Sorghum bicolor* (L.) Moench] and millet (*Panicum miliaceum* L.) are other cereals upon which large numbers of the world's people also depend for daily sustenance. Because of their importance the cereals, particularly wheat, will be examined in this presentation.

The major cereal food species are consumed in the form of food products prepared from their seed. The cereals are perceived by most people as carbohydrate foods but they are important sources of protein, minerals, and vitamins as well. The relative nutritional value of the

[1] Presented at symposium on "Crops as Sources of Nutrients for Humans". Annual meetings, Am. Soc. of Agron., 2 Dec. 1982, Anaheim, CA.

[2] Leader wheat research, USDA, ARS, Lincoln, NE.

cereals is determined largely by the amount and kind of storage proteins contained in their seed.

Food plant species differ widely in the amount and quality of their protein (4). The legumes are notably high in amounts of protein; the cereals contain much lower amounts, and the root crops the least. Few if any of the plant species produce protein with nutritional quality comparable to that of meat, milk, and other animal products. Plant storage proteins seldom contain essential amino acids in the relative amounts required for maximum utilization of the protein by man and monogastric animals. The plant proteins differ as well in their digestibility and availability.

The cornerstone of breeding improvement of the crop species is availability of useable genetic variation. If such genetic variation does not occur naturally in a species it must be induced or it must be transferred from related species if breeding improvement is to take place. The genetic complexity of the trait being manipulated, genetic linkages with other traits, phenotypic expression, ease of observation or measurement of the trait and relative magnitude of genetic and nongenetic effects also contribute significantly to the success of the plant breeding effort.

Because of their importance as food species and their projected contribution to increased future world food production, the cereals, particularly wheat, rice, maize, and sorghum, have undergone intensive research to improve their nutritional value by breeding. The research has focused on improved protein quality as well as increased amount of protein. Research emphasis in each species has been strongly influenced by the particular nutritional deficiencies of the species as well as by availability of useable genetic variation. Among the four most important food cereals, maize and sorghum have the poorest quality protein. Rice has the best quality. Wheat is intermediate in protein quality but it normally has a higher concentration of protein in its grain than the other three major cereals. Sorghum has the added problem of tannins and other organic compounds that interfere with the availability and digestibility of its protein.

BREEDING FOR IMPROVED QUALITY OF PROTEIN

Genes that significantly enhance the nutritional quality of maize, sorghum, and barley (*Hordeum vulgare* L.) have been identified. In each case, the genes increase the concentration of the essential amino acid lysine, thereby resulting in protein that more nearly provides the essential amino acids in the amounts required by humans and other monogastric animals. The *opaque-2* gene in maize also significantly increases a second essential amino acid tryptophan.

In wheat and rice, there has been little progress to date in genetic improvement of protein quality. Genes with large effect on level of lysine have not been found in either species. It should be pointed out that protein quality improvement in rice and wheat is not perceived to be as critical as it is in maize and sorghum because each has better quality protein than the latter two (4). According to nutritionists, even ordinary wheat, with poorer quality protein than rice, if consumed in sufficient quantity to satisfy caloric requirements of people, will also provide enough protein and essential amino acids to meet nutritional requirements, except for pregnant or lactating women and very young children.

In each of the cereals in which major genes for improved protein quality have been identified, the improvement results from an altered ratio of protein fractions in which the lysine-poor fraction constitutes a smaller proportion of total protein in the grain. In cereals, the prolamine fraction is notably poor in lysine. A second similarity of the genes is their adverse effect on seed density and texture and on grain yield. Any reduction of grain yield to achieve nutritional quality enhancement is perceived by scientists and producers as unacceptable. Consequently, the acceptance and use of high lysine maize, sorghum, and barley has been much slower than initially anticipated and awaits the development of high quality varieties and hybrids that are fully competitive in yield with currently grown types. Although substantial progress already has been made toward that end, nutritionally improved types continue to comprise an extremely small part of total world production of the three crops.

Useable genetic variation for protein and lysine in rice may have been recently demonstrated (3). Genetic engineering techniques were employed by ARS scientists at Beltsville, Md. to develop rice plants that produce more protein with higher lysine concentration than ordinary rice. Doubled haploid plants propagated from cell clumps in undifferentiated callus tissue from rice anther culture were found to produce seed containing above normal concentrations of protein and lysine. Research is currently under way to ascertain the inheritance of the increased protein and lysine, and the degree to which the effect can be transferred to high yielding, agronomically acceptable rice varieties. The potential of this and other tissue culture techniques for nutritional improvement of the other cereals is not known.

Genetic control of lysine in wheat protein has been demonstrated by Nebraska research (2, 6, 8). We have identified genes that influence lysine content of wheat protein, but the magnitude of the increase is small compared with that needed to bring lysine into balance with other essential amino acids. Also, production environment and concentration of protein in the seed influence lysine content of the protein and add to the difficulty of genetic manipulation of lysine in a breeding program.

IMPROVEMENT OF PROTEIN QUANTITY OF WHEAT
BY BREEDING

In contrast to the limited genetic variation for lysine in wheat, substantial genetic variation for protein has been uncovered (6, 7, 8, 11). We have identified genes in the 'Atlas 66' and 'Atlas 50' cultivars and in 'Nap Hal'. At least one of two genes for protein in Atlas 66 was transferred in Nebraska to the productive leaf rust-resistant hard red winter wheat cv. Lancota (7, 10). A similar transfer of genes for elevated protein from Atlas

50 to experimental lines of hard red winter wheat was accomplished at Kansas State Univ. (9).

Genes for high grain protein in *Aegilops* were transferred to the hard red winter cvs. Plainsman V and Century II by a private seed company in Kansas. Plants have been identified among collections of wild-growing *Triticum dicoccoides* in Israel that produce larger-than-normal seed with significantly higher protein content than the other *T. dicoccoides* collections. Research is in progress in Israel to determine the degree to which the elevated protein trait found in *T. dicoccoides* can be transferred to cultivated wheat. Evidence of the presence of minor genes in common wheat varieties has been demonstrated (5).

We combined the high protein genes in Atlas 66 and Nap Hal by hybridization and produced progeny lines in which grain protein content as much as 5 percentage points higher than ordinary wheat was achieved. Because the initial high protein lines were nonproductive, tall, small seeded, agronomically unacceptable and had undesirable processing qualities, it could not be established whether protein improvement was compatible with high productivity and other necessary agronomic and quality traits or whether it was mainly an artifact of nonproductivity.

Results from second and third breeding cycles involving the Atlas 66 × Nap Hal and other high protein combinations at Nebraska provide reassuring evidence of the compatibility of high protein with other important traits in wheat. The performance of six high protein lines grown in a 60-entry replicated irrigated winter wheat nursery at Yuma, Ariz. in 1982 is compared with the check cv. TAM 105 in Table 1. Three of the lines were significantly more productive, produced significantly larger seed, and were significantly higher in protein content than TAM 105. All but one line had straw as short or shorter than TAM 105. The grain yield and protein content of all 60 lines in the trial are plotted in Fig. 1. Those encircled were equal to TAM 105 in yield but significantly higher in protein content. Dough development properties of selected high protein lines as measured by the mixograph and shown in Fig. 2 reveal a wide range in mixing characteristics.

Seventy high protein spring wheats also were evaluated at Yuma in 1982. None was significantly higher yielding than Super X in a replicated irrigated trial but 22 were equal to Super X in yield and were significantly higher in grain protein content (Fig. 3). The performance of eight promising lines summarized in Table 2 provides strong evidence that high grain protein can be combined with large seed and short straw in high yielding wheats. Mixographs shown in Fig. 4 reveal a wide range in types similar to that found among the high protein winter wheats.

BREEDING CONSTRAINTS

The protein content of wheat and other cereals is strongly influenced by grain yield. This negative relationship is particularly pronounced in favorable production areas in which availability of soil N is limited. In these areas, use of cultivars or hybrids with potential for high grain yield may result in high yields of grain with depressed protein content. This has

Table 1. Performance of promising high protein winter wheat lines in replicated
irrigated trials, Yuma, Ariz., 1982.

Entry	Maturity†	Plant height‡	100-seed weight	Grain yield	Grain protein§
			g	kg/ha	%
33	ME	MS	3.5	6460	13.3
28	E	Med	4.3	5275	16.3
24	E	S	3.8	5040	16.2
35	E	MS	3.9	4855	15.6
25	E	S	4.0	4540	16.1
27	E	MS	3.8	4115	18.2
TAM 105	ML	MS	3.1	3700	13.0
LSD$_{0.05}$	--	--	0.5	990	2.0

† ME = moderately early, E = early, ML = moderately late.
‡ MS = moderately short, Med. = medium, S = short.
§ Dry weight basis.

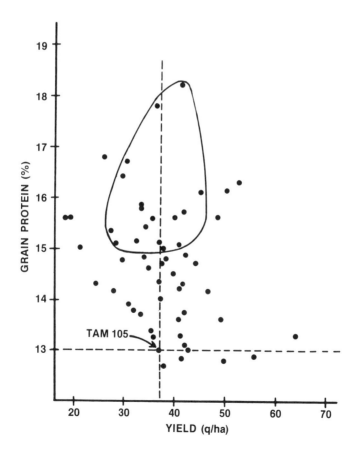

Fig. 1. Yield of high protein winter wheats grown in replicated irrigated trials at Yuma, Ariz., 1982.

influenced some breeders to reject protein improvement as a viable breeding objective. In wheat it is doubtful that protein depression frequently associated with high yields can be entirely overcome in all environments. Accumulated data suggest that the depression can be effectively reduced and, in some production environments, actually reversed by incorporating high protein genes into productive cultivars.

A second constraint results from the tendency for protein concentration to be negatively correlated with lysine concentration of the protein

Table 2. Performance of promising high protein spring wheat lines in replicated irrigated trials, Yuma, Ariz., 1982.

Entry	Maturity†	Plant height‡	100-seed weight	Grain yield	Grain protein§
			g	kg/ha	%
15	L	MT	3.8	6210	15.6
5	Med	MS	2.8	6163	16.2
17	ME	Med	5.0	5816	15.8
7	ML	Med	3.2	5670	16.8
33	E	S	4.6	5143	16.9
31	ME	MS	4.4	5127	16.4
42	E	MS	3.7	5110	16.7
35	E	S	3.1	4897	17.8
Super X	E	S	4.3	5257	13.2
LSD$_{0.05}$	--	--	0.4	1090	1.5

† L = late, Med = medium, ME = moderately early, ML = moderately late, E = early.
‡ MT = moderately tall, MS = moderately short, Med = medium, S = short.
§ Dry weight basis.

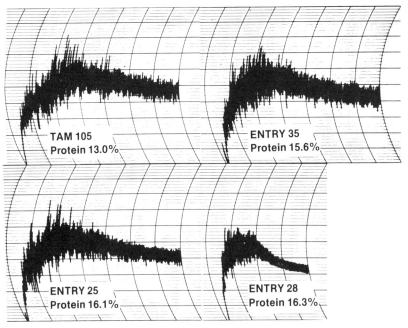

Fig. 2. Mixograms of high protein winter wheat lines.

(6). In wheat, the depression results from altered ratios of protein fractions with changes in concentration of seed protein. The proportion of lysine-poor gliadin increases with higher protein concentration. The negative relationship of lysine and protein in wheat is most pronounced at levels of protein up to approximately 15%. Protein differences above the 15% level have been found to have little further effect on lysine concentration. Despite the depression of lysine per unit of protein associated with elevated protein content of wheat seed, lysine per unit grain weight increases with protein level. Therefore, high protein wheat can be expected to contain more lysine than lower protein wheat.

Bioenergy implications of changing the concentration of cereal grain protein has been suggested as a further constraint to breeding for high protein in wheat. Researchers at the International Atomic Energy Agency calculated that increased inputs of carbon assimilates and N would be needed to increase protein concentration in cereal grains while maintaining high grain yields (1). Presumably, such enhanced inputs would be increasingly difficult to achieve when high yielding wheats are grown in

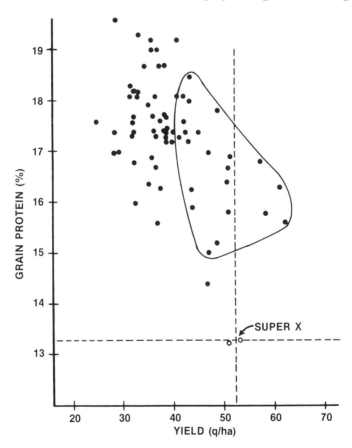

Fig. 3. Yield of high protein spring wheats grown in replicated irrigated trials at Yuma, Ariz., 1982.

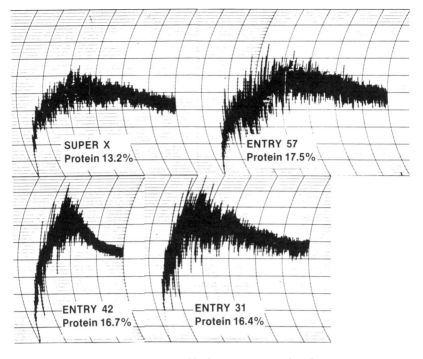

Fig. 4. Mixograms of high protein spring wheat lines.

favorable production environments that permit maximum expression of their genetic potential for high yield. There is little agreement among breeders about the reality of the suggested bioenergy constraints in most production environments. Much of the world's wheat is produced in rainfed areas in which powerful environmental constraints limit yields and interfere with full expression of genetic yield potential. In such suboptimal production environments the calculated increased bioenergy requirements of high protein wheat may not constitute a breeding barrier.

For many cereal breeders throughout the world, the most serious constraint to breeding for higher protein may be the lack of laboratory facilities for rapid protein analyses of large numbers of experimental lines commonly associated with early stages of breeding. When the breeder is forced to relegate selection for protein to secondary status to be performed at late stages of the breeding process when the number of lines to be analyzed is less, the likelihood of progress is greatly diminished.

PROTEIN SEPARATION BY SEED FLOTATION

We are currently evaluating an inexpensive simple system for separating wheat seed on the basis of its protein content. The technique, which was developed by Mr. A. Garzon Trula, Office of the Director General for Farm Production, Ministry of Agriculture in Madrid, Spain and reported in a study entitled "Basics of Seed Densimetry" in 1981, is based on solvent flotation. Starch density of wheat is 1.6 g/ml compared with protein density of 1.2 g/ml. Protein absorbs approximately five times more H_2O than starch when the seed is soaked in H_2O for 7 to 10 days. If the soaking is done at 0 to 1°C germination is inhibited and the seed remains viable. Following soaking, high protein seed can be separated from lower protein seed in a solvent solution of carbon tetrachloride and hexane with density of approximately 1.25 (Fig. 5) H_2O presoaking prevents the solvent from penetrating the seed and interfering with germination. Following separation the seed fractions can be airdried without loss of viability and subsequently planted normally. Germination of air dried high protein seed following solvent separation is shown in Fig. 6.

We believe the technique has exciting possibilities for inexpensively recovering high protein seed from bulk hybrid populations known to be segregating for protein. The only apparatus required for the procedure is a small chamber in which temperature can be controlled at 0 to 1°C and ventilated hood to remove solvent fumes during flotation. The technique also requires that shrivelled kernels be removed from the bulk since these would separate with the high protein fraction and are not likely to be

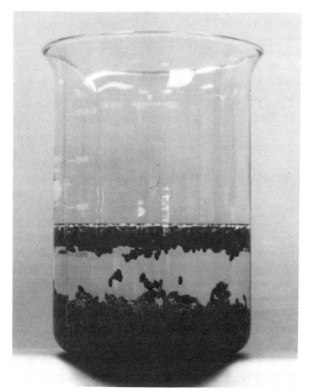

Fig. 5. High protein seed with density less than that of the solvent solution, floats while the lower protein seed remains at the bottom of the container.

Table 3. Separation of high protein from low protein wheat seed in bulk hybrids
by solvent flotation.

	Protein content (%)	
Population	High protein fraction	Low protein fraction
Exp'l Hybrid 1	19.0	16.1
Exp'l Hybrid 2	18.1	16.3
Exp'l Hybrid 3	17.2	15.2
Exp'l Hybrid 4	18.6	13.8
Exp'l Hybrid 5	17.4	14.3
Exp'l Hybrid 6	18.1	15.0
Lancota (check)	14.3	12.5

Based on method of Mr. A. Garzon Trula, Ministry of Agriculture, Madrid, Spain.

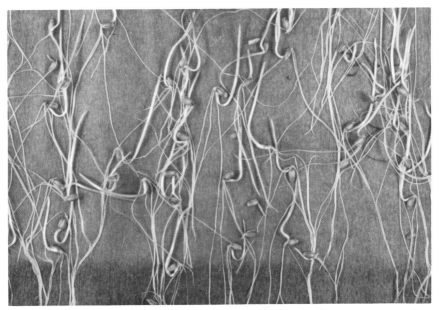

Fig. 6. High protein seed, retrieved by solvent flotation and air dried, germinates normally.

genetically high in protein. The efficiency of separation is shown in Table
3. Carbon tetrachloride must be handled with care to avoid dangerous
contact with the liquid and fumes. Currently we are seeking an alternative solvent with similar but safer properties for use in the procedure. We
have not determined the effectiveness of the technique for seed separation
on the basis of protein content in other cereals.

REFERENCES

1. Bhatia, C. R., and R. Rabson. 1976. Bio-energetic consideration in cereal breeding for
   protein improvement. Science 194:1418–1421.
2. Diehl, A. L., V. A. Johnson, and P. J. Mattern. 1978. Inheritance of protein and lysine
   in three wheat crosses. Crop Sci. 17:391–395.

3. Genetic Engineering in Agriculture. 1982. Test tube rice yields better protein. AR, USDA, September 1982. p. 14.

4. Johnson, V. A., and C. L. Lay. 1974. Genetic improvement of plant protein. J. Agric. Food Chem. 22:558–566.

5. ----, and P. J. Mattern. 1980. Genetic improvement of productivity and nutritional quality of wheat. Final Report of Research Findings. Contract No. AID/csd-1208 and AID/ta-c-1903. USDA-SEA-ARS and Univ. of Nebraska, IANR. 110 p.

6. ----, ----, J. W. Schmidt, and J. E. Stroike. 1973. Genetic advances in wheat protein quantity and composition. p. 547–556. *In* Proc. 4th Int. Wheat Gen. Symp. Missouri Agric. Exp. Stn., Columbia, MO 1973.

7. ----, ----, K. D. Wilhelmi, and S. L. Kuhr. 1977. Seed protein improvement in common wheat (*Triticum aestivum* L.): opportunities and constraints. Proc. Int. Conf. on Seed Protein Improvement by Nuclear Techniques, Baden, Austria, 1977. IAEA-RC-57/2:23–32.

8. ----, K. D. Wilhelmi, S. L. Kuhr, P. J. Mattern, and J. W. Schmidt. 1978. Breeding progress for protein and lysine in wheat. p. 825–835. *In* Proc. 5th Int. Wheat Gen. Symp. New Delhi, India, 1978.

9. Miezan, K., E. G. Heyne, and K. F. Finney. 1977. Genetic and environmental effects on grain protein content in wheat. Crop Sci. 17:591–593.

10. Schmidt, J. W., V. A. Johnson, P. J. Mattern, A. F. Dreier, and D. V. McVey. 1979. Registration of Lancota wheat. Crop Sci. 19:749.

11. Vogel, K. P., V. A. Johnson, and P. J. Mattern. 1978. Protein and lysine contents of endosperm and bran of the parents and progenies of crosses of common wheat. Crop Sci. 18:751–754.